Management and Administration for the OTA

Leadership and Application Skills

Management and Administration for the OTA

Leadership and Application Skills

EDITOR

KAREN JACOBS, EDD, OTR/L, CPE, FAOTA

CLINICAL PROFESSOR & PROGRAM DIRECTOR

DISTANCE EDUCATION POST-PROFESSIONAL DOCTORATE IN OCCUPATIONAL THERAPY PROGRAM

BOSTON UNIVERSITY COLLEGE OF HEALTH AND REHABILITATION SCIENCES: SARGENT COLLEGE

DEPARTMENT OF OCCUPATIONAL THERAPY

BOSTON, MASSACHUSETTS

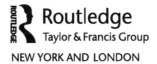

Routledge
Taylor & Francis Group

NEW YORK AND LONDON

Instructors: *Management and Administration for the OTA: Leadership and Application Skills Instructor's Manual* is also available. Don't miss this important companion to *Management and Administration for the OTA: Leadership and Application Skills*. To obtain the Instructor's Manual, please visit http://www.routledge.com/9781630910655

First published in 2016 SLACK Incorporated

Published 2024 by Routledge
605 Third Avenue, New York, NY 10158

and by Routledge
4 Park Square, Milton Park, Abingdon, Oxon OX14 4RN

Routledge is an imprint of the Taylor & Francis Group, an informa business

Library of Congress Cataloging-in-Publication Data

Management and administration for the OTA : leadership and application skills / [edited by] Karen Jacobs.
    p. ; cm.
  Includes bibliographical references and index.
  ISBN 9781630910655 (alk. paper)
  I. Jacobs, Karen, editor.
  [DNLM: 1. Occupational Therapy--organization & administration. 2. Leadership. WB 555]
  RM735
  615.8'515--dc23
                     2015012443

ISBN: 9781630910655 (pbk)
ISBN: 9781003524939 (ebk)

DOI: 10.4324/9781003524939

Additional resources can be found at https:// www.routledge.com/9781630910655

DEDICATION

To my parents, who have always been the wind beneath my wings, and to my children and grandchildren, who help me live life to its fullest.

CONTENTS

ACKNOWLEDGMENTS

Thank you to all the authors who wrote the chapters contained in this book. It was a pleasure working with you. Much appreciation is shared with SLACK Incorporated, especially John, Brien, April, Kirstin, and Trevor.

ABOUT THE EDITOR

Karen Jacobs, EdD, OTR/L, CPE, FAOTA, is a clinical professor of occupational therapy and the program director of the online post-professional doctorate in occupational therapy program at Boston University. She has worked at Boston University for 31 years and has expertise in the development and instruction of online graduate courses.

Karen earned a doctoral degree at the University of Massachusetts, a master of science degree from Boston University, and a bachelor of arts degree from Washington University in St. Louis, Missouri.

Karen is a past president and vice president of the American Occupational Therapy Association. She is a 2005 recipient of a Fulbright Scholarship to the University of Akureyri in Akuryeri, Iceland. Karen also received the 2009 Award of Merit from the Canadian Association of Occupational Therapists; the Award of Merit from the American Occupational Therapy Association in 2003; and the 2011 Eleanor Clarke Slagle Lectureship Award. The title of her Slagle Lecture was "PromOTing Occupational Therapy: Words, Images, and Action."

In addition to being an occupational therapist, Karen is also a certified professional ergonomist and the founding editor-in-chief of the international, interprofessional journal *WORK: A Journal of Prevention, Assessment & Rehabilitation* (IOS Press, The Netherlands) and is a consultant in ergonomics, marketing, and entrepreneurship.

CONTRIBUTING AUTHORS

Karen Brady, DEd, OTR/L (Chapter 3)
Assistant Professor
Department of Occupational Therapy
Panuska College of Professional Studies
The University of Scranton
Scranton, Pennsylvania

Lisa Burns, PhD, OTR/L (Chapter 3)
Assistant Professor
Murphy Deming College of Health Sciences
Mary Baldwin College
Fishersville, Virginia

Nancy W. Doyle, OTD, OTR/L (Chapter 9)
Lecturer
Department of Occupational Therapy
Boston University
Boston, Massachusetts

Kimberly Erler, MS, OTR/L (Chapter 10)
Massachusetts General Hospital
Boston, Massachusetts

Brenda Kennell, BS, MA, OTR/L (Chapter 6)
Program Director
Occupational Therapy Assistant Program
Central Piedmont Community College
Charlotte, North Carolina

Barbara Larson, MA, OTR/L, FAOTA (Chapter 4)
Independent Consultation, Work and Industry
Adjunct Faculty and On-Campus Clinic Director
Occupational Therapy Program
The College of St. Scholastica
Duluth, Minnesota

Ann McCullough, BA (Chapter 1)
Occupational Therapy Student
Boston University
Boston, Massachusetts

Sarah McKinnon, MS, OTR/L (Chapter 2)
Adjunct Faculty
Department of Occupational Therapy
Boston University
Boston, Massachusetts

Julie Ann Nastasi, ScD, OTD, OTR/L, SCLV, FAOTA (Chapter 8)
Faculty Specialist
Department of Occupational Therapy
The University of Scranton
Scranton, Pennsylvania

Linda Niemeyer, OT, PhD (Chapter 11)
Lecturer in Occupational Therapy
Sargent College of Health and Rehabilitation Sciences
Department of Occupational Therapy
Boston University
Boston, Massachusetts

Melissa J. Tilton, BS, COTA/L, ROH (Foreword)
Clinical Operations Area Director
Genesis Rehab
Saugus, Massachusetts

Christi Vicino, MA, OTA/L (Chapter 7)
Occupational Therapy Assistant
Program Director
Grossmont College
El Cajon, California

FOREWORD

When I was first asked to write the foreword for *Management and Administration for the OTA: Leadership and Application Skills*, I was giddy with excitement and I thought, "Who, me?" What an honor, as an occupational therapy assistant (OTA), to share my admiration for this book and for the editor, as well as to promote the role of an OTA. Dr. Jacobs and I have been friends for years now and this friendship blossomed out of a mutual admiration for volunteerism and being part of the occupational therapy (OT) community. I first met her while organizing our state OT association conference committee meetings. We truly gelled when Dr. Jacobs asked me to come and speak to her master's-level occupational therapist students about reimbursement. Dr. Jacobs proudly, but sincerely, introduced me (at that time) as the President of MAOT, a knowledgeable lecturer, and an experienced and active OTA. She wanted the students to learn and wanted them to understand that growth comes in learning from all, despite their title. This action, for me, demonstrated her belief and her practice, in having a partnership and collaboration between the OT and OTA, and her true passion for self-improvement, in order to help those we work with to better themselves. I continue to work with Dr. Jacobs to bring up-to-date information to her students, to demonstrate the value of the OT/OTA collaboration, and to continue to advance my own leadership skills—all of which I am humbly grateful for.

Leadership, volunteerism, and advocacy is at the heart of what I do as an OTA; it is what keeps me going and fills my bucket. Knowing that OTAs have the skill set and the opportunity to lead is vital to our profession. In Chapter 2, OTAs are encouraged to become involved, to identify their leadership style, and to have a purposeful outcome. The reader is provided with examples of leadership opportunities in their own community, whether it be in their state or nationally. However, to take that next step into leadership, the reader will learn the importance of marketing and how they complete a SWOT analysis, in order to move forward. Sometimes we are not sure where to start, but this helps get us going. Having the ability to understand your values, your strengths, and knowing where you want to go will continue to support the advancement of OTAs as valued team members in the OT field.

"Supervision of the OTA is a two-way street" (p. 93). I love this quote! As an OTA, we also need supervision, and should want supervision. Dr. Jacobs' book provides an explanation of the varied levels of supervision, from entry-level to the experienced OTA, and an understanding of how we may move through these levels based on our competency or enter new areas of practice. The heart of the matter is summed up quite well—we need to have supervision and the process is "a cooperative process" (p. 93). We need to have meaningful supervision and collaboration, we need to give and receive, and we need to share ideas and brainstorm together. We need to utilize this process in a heartfelt manner, ensuring that the good of the client is our joint focus, while encouraging growth and continued competency.

Scholarly activities and involvement is an area of opportunity for OTAs. The how, the why, the application, are all areas we are competent in. However, understanding the impact of, the use of, how this use of scholarly information can change outcomes, and how this relates to healthcare reform and reimbursement are crucial for the future of our practice. Additionally, as OTAs, the possibility of involvement in scholarly activities is our responsibility and privilege! We need to understand this information and apply this information in our everyday practice arenas. For the newer OTA, Chapter 11 clearly explains the differences between qualitative and quantitative research and provides an easy-to-use tool on the criteria for trustworthy research in both research styles. This book shows us the entry-level information, but also the tools to move forward and challenge ourselves in staying current with the trends in occupational therapy.

While there are too many parts of this book to share with you in this little-bitty foreword, I encourage you to dive in, soak it all up, and share what you learn with your colleagues and students. Identify how you can use this newly gained knowledge in your everyday world to encourage you to lead, to grow, to advocate, to achieve better outcomes, and to live life to the fullest.

—Melissa J. Tilton, BS, COTA/L, ROH
Vice President of the Massachusetts Association for Occupational Therapy
Saugus, Massachusetts

INTRODUCTION

"Never doubt that a small group of thoughtful, concerned citizens can change the world. Indeed, it is the only thing that ever has."

—Margaret Mead

The 11 chapters in *Management and Administration for the OTA: Leadership and Application Skills* address all of the 2011 Accreditation Council for Occupational Therapy Education standards for an associate degree educational program for an occupational therapy assistant (OTA) related to management, administration, and leadership. The chapters were ably authored by occupational therapy professionals with varied backgrounds: clinicians, academicians, administrators, managers, graduate students; and many have instructed or worked with OTAs in different contexts.

The book begins with the chapter on *Contexts and Health Care*, which addresses the contexts of health care and the potential impact of policy issues as they relate to the practice of occupational therapy. Chapter 2 is about *Leadership and Advocacy*; these are two important roles that we all need to take on to be agents of change. *Credentialing* is the focus of Chapter 3, which introduces the national requirements for credentialing and for licensure, certification, or registration under state laws. Chapter 4 is about *Reimbursement*. This chapter explains the various reimbursement system requirements that affect the practice of occupational therapy. Chapter 5 is on *Marketing and Promoting*; it is our responsibility to promote the distinct value of occupational therapy to the public (individuals, groups, and populations), as well as to other professionals, service providers, consumers, third-party payers, and regulatory bodies. Chapter 6 discusses *Documentation and Quality Improvement* to ensure that we provide the highest quality of occupational therapy services. Chapter 7 provides information about *Supervision*—it also helps us to understand the important relationship between the OTA, the occupational therapist, and nonprofessional personnel. Chapter 8 describes the ongoing professional responsibility of *Fieldwork*. Chapter 9 helps us have a better understanding of *Communication Skills: Health Literacy*. We must all demonstrate knowledge and understanding of the American Occupational Therapy Association's (AOTA's) *Occupational Therapy Code of Ethics and Ethics Standards*, as well as the AOTA *Standards of Practice*, which is introduced in Chapter 10. Finally, the book concludes with Chapter 11 on *The Importance of Scholarship and Scholarly Practice for the OTA*, which will help you articulate the important contribution of scholarly activities and evidence-based literature to the distinct value and advancement of occupational therapy. Each chapter contains website resources, multiple-choice questions, and thoughtful case examples that help the content come alive.

It was a pleasure being the editor of this textbook and I thank all of the authors for their contributions and SLACK Incorporated for their support in making *Management and Administration for the OTA: Leadership and Application Skills* a reality.

—Karen Jacobs, EdD, OTR/L, CPE, FAOTA

Contexts and Health Care

Ann McCullough, BA

Accreditation Council for Occupational Therapy Education (ACOTE) Standards explored in this chapter are the following:

- B.6.1. Describe the contexts of health care, education, community, and social systems as they relate to the practice of occupational therapy.

- B.6.2. Identify the potential impact of current policy issues and the social, economic, political, geographic, or demographic factors on the practice of occupational therapy.

- B.7.1. Identify the impact of contextual factors on the management and delivery of occupational therapy services.

- B.7.2. Identify the systems and structures that create federal and state legislation and regulations and their implications and effects on practice.

KEY VOCABULARY

Entitlement: Legislation that guarantees rights to benefits to specific groups of individuals.

Medicare: Federal insurance program for individuals over 65 years old or with specific conditions.

Medicaid: Federal-state partnership meant to provide health insurance to some groups of individuals who cannot afford insurance.

Habilitative services: Health care services that help a person keep, learn, or improve skills and functioning for daily living.

Telehealth: Electronic information and telecommunication to support long-distance health care and health administration.

Jacobs K, ed.
Management and Administration for the OTA:
Leadership and Application Skills (pp 1-14).
© 2016 Taylor & Francis Group.

CASE STUDY

Ruth is an 80-year-old woman living in Chicago with her 56-year-old daughter and son-in-law. She was in good health until 2 weeks ago, when she was in a minor car accident during which she broke her right arm and leg. Her 25-year-old grandson, Dave, was in the car as well and suffered a concussion. You have just started seeing her in an outpatient clinic. Although she is making significant progress, she is frequently confused about her health insurance information, and is concerned about what type of care her grandson will be able to receive. You have referred her to a social worker who is working with her to ensure that she and her family receive all the benefits to which they are entitled. However, you would like to better understand the rules and regulations that affect her and her access to occupational therapy services.

Throughout this chapter, you will learn more about how the experiences of people like Ruth and Dave are affected by specific historical and social contexts, including legislation, policy issues, geography, and demographics. Similarly, the experiences of occupational therapy practitioners are also shaped by these contexts because they impact where and how practitioners work, how they are reimbursed, and which clients have access to occupational therapy services. Examining the history of legislation in health care, education, and social systems that has impacted the practice of occupational therapy demonstrates how occupational therapy is shaped by specific contexts. The history of these policies also provides insight into how the most recent legislative changes may impact occupational therapy in the near future and how new legislation may be created.

ENTITLEMENT LEGISLATION

Much of the legislation that addresses health care, education, and social systems falls under the category of entitlement. Entitlement can be defined as laws that guarantee rights to benefits to specific groups of individuals (Freedman, 2012). Some examples include Social Security, Medicare, Medicaid, Children's Health Insurance Program (CHIP), Supplemental Nutrition Assistance Program, Individuals with Disabilities Education Act (IDEA), and, most recently, the Patient Protection and Affordable Care Act (ACA; Pub. L. 111-148). Other legislation that impacts the practice of occupational therapy includes the Americans with Disabilities Act (ADA) and various budgets.

Social Security Act

The Social Security Act is the oldest of these legislations. This act was passed by President Franklin D. Roosevelt in 1935 during the time of the Great Depression, when many people in the United States were experiencing financial difficulties. The act laid the foundation for future laws and reforms in the areas of health care, education, community, and social systems and included early versions of many policies that are still in place today. The act included federal grants to states for programs to help those who were perceived as most in need at the time: Federal Old-Age, Survivors, Disability, and Hospital Insurance; Old Age Assistance; programs to aid individuals who were blind; programs to aid dependent children; Maternal and Child Health; Crippled Children Services; vocational rehabilitation; and Child Welfare Services. It avoided any mention of state or national health insurance (Cohen, 1983). The passage of the Social Security Act was dependent on compromise between the political positions of many different groups, including those who wanted to maintain the professional autonomy of physicians and those who wanted health care benefits to remain linked to employment and union membership (Rothman, 2005). Without a national or state health insurance program, private health insurance became a reasonable option for most members of the middle class. Blue Cross health insurance was a hospital-based insurance developed in 1929 that established a third-party payment system and shaped future private health insurance (Lohman, 2014). During World War II, advances in medical care, technology, and medicine caused increases in the cost of health care. Enrollment in private and nonprofit health insurance occurred between 1940 and 1945 to help people pay for expensive treatments (Parks, 2012). During this time, private insurance remained unaffordable for many people who did not receive insurance from their employers, shaping the debate around government-sponsored insurance programs.

Many health care reforms have been implemented since 1935. These reforms have primarily addressed three concerns: cost, access, and quality. Many policymakers and analysts argue that these factors create an "iron triangle" because they are interdependent and in competition with each other (Mehta & Jha, 2012). Improving one or two of these areas causes a negative impact on the third area. For example, if a reform focuses on reducing costs, it may also be possible to increase access to those who could not afford health care before. However, such a change will likely decrease the quality of care because each client will have access to fewer resources. This "iron triangle" demonstrates why continuous reform is both necessary and difficult since each reform often creates new challenges that need to be addressed. Occupational therapy practitioners are concerned with each of these three factors because they all affect the experiences of our clients and impact the practice of occupational therapy.

Medicare

Medicare came out of the same discussion of national health insurance that began before the passage of the Social Security Act. President Harry S. Truman pushed for national health insurance during his terms in office, from 1945 to 1953. Although Congress did not pass a health insurance law, President Truman's proposal kept alive a national debate about health care reform. Since President Truman was unsuccessful in convincing Congress to pass a law for national health insurance, his supporters proposed that a focus on older adults might be more successful politically (Kronenfeld, 2011). The elderly were widely perceived as a sympathetic group. Many Americans could relate to this group and could expect to be a part of it one day. Furthermore, since health insurance was mostly provided through the workplace at the time, people past retirement age were more likely to be uninsured. Medicare was passed into law in 1965 under President Lyndon B. Johnson. The initial law was created as an insurance program for individuals over the age of 65 and included only Part A to cover hospital services and Part B to cover outpatient services, including occupational therapy.

Between 1965 and 2010, Medicare received many expansions and revisions. Lohman (2014) outlined how these reforms impacted the practice of occupational therapy. The passage of Medicare provided more people with access to occupational therapy services, thus encouraging the growth of occupational therapy practice. In 1972, Medicare was extended to people under the age of 65 with disabilities and end-stage renal disease, extending occupational therapy services to these populations. Some additional reforms included or excluded occupational therapy as a qualifying service in various settings, placed limits on how many visits would be reimbursed, and defined how clients could qualify for services. In 1981, the Budget Reconciliation Act eliminated occupational therapy as a qualifying service with home health, thus requiring that nursing, speech therapy, or physical therapy qualify a client for skilled care. Being recognized as a qualifying service with home health is still an issue that we face today. More occupational therapy practitioners began working in hospice and in skilled nursing facilities after a 1982 reform enacted hospice benefits, and a 1983 reform reduced the length of stay in acute impatient settings.

The current Medicare coverage is as follows:

- Population covered:
  - Those 65 years of age or older, U.S. citizens or residents for over 5 years, who have paid (or spouse has paid) Medicare taxes for the past 10 years.
  - Those younger than 65 years of age with a permanent disability who have received Social Security disability benefits for the past 2 years.
  - Those younger than 65 years of ago who receive Social Security disability benefits for amyotrophic lateral sclerosis (ALS).
  - Those younger than 65 years of age who need continuous dialysis or a kidney transplant (Askin & Moore, 2012).
- Parts:
  - **Part A** covers inpatient services, including stays in hospitals and skilled nursing facilities, home health visits, and hospice.
  - **Part B** covers outpatient services, including visits to physicians and other health care providers, preventative services, home health visits, and durable medical equipment.
  - **Part C** (also called Medicare Advantage) provides an option for beneficiaries to purchase insurance from a private company which contracts with Medicare to provide all Part A and Part B benefits, and may provide additional benefits. Medicare pays private insurers a fixed amount each month, per beneficiary.
  - **Part D** provides outpatient prescription drug coverage through private plans that contract with Medicare. (Askin & Moore, 2012)

Both Part C and Part D are voluntary programs. Medicare Part A and Part B do not cover all services that the population it serves may need. For example, it does not cover long-term custodial care, routine dental and eye care, dentures, cosmetic surgery, acupuncture, hearing aids, and routine foot care. Medicare includes many restrictions and limits, such as the number of days that are covered for inpatient stays, the number of visits to a physician or therapist, and specific services that are reimbursed. Since Medicare is the largest payer of health care in the United States, its policies influence how health care, including occupational therapy services, is provided overall (Lohman, 2014).

Medicaid

Medicaid was passed into law in 1965 by President Lyndon B. Johnson at the same time as Medicare. Unlike Medicare, Medicaid is a federal-state partnership, and states can elect whether to participate. States receive most of the funding for Medicaid money from the federal government, but programs are regulated by each state. To receive federal funding, states must cover individuals who are in the following "categorically eligible" groups whose income is 20% less than the federal poverty level: children, parents with dependent children, pregnant women, people with severe disabilities, and seniors. Seniors older than the age of 65 may already be enrolled in Medicare, but can receive Medicaid to help cover premiums, out-of-pocket medical expenses, and other services not covered by Medicare. States may also decide to cover additional classes of individuals or may decide to have a higher income threshold for eligibility. At a minimum, states are required to provide coverage for the following:

- Inpatient and outpatient hospital services
- Physician, midwife, and nurse practitioner services
- Laboratory and x-ray services

- Nursing facility services and home health care for individuals aged 21 years and older
- Early and periodic screening, diagnosis, and treatment for children younger than 2 years of age
- Family planning services and supplies
- Rural health clinic and federally qualified health center services (Askin & Moore, 2012)

Individual states may decide to provide additional coverage. Since Medicaid law allows states to regulate the eligibility and coverage, significant differences may exist among states. Occupational therapy is considered an optional service under Medicaid, so states can choose whether to cover occupational therapy services. However, a state must reimburse occupational therapy services if a child is covered under the Early and Periodic Screening, Diagnosis, and Treatment (EPSDT) benefit and a physician has ordered occupational therapy as medically necessary (Lohman, 2014). Similar to Medicare, Medicaid policies have far-reaching impacts on health care services in the United States because Medicaid covers one-quarter of all children in the United States and two-thirds of all nursing home residents (Lohman, 2014).

CHIP is part of a state's Medicaid program, and was established in 1997. The purpose of this program is to expand the coverage of Medicaid to provide coverage to children who are not eligible for Medicaid. The specific regulations and coverage are decided by each state, although the benefits are similar to those under Medicaid. Coverage may include limits in services or deductibles.

The Patient Protection and Affordable Care Act

The most recent health care reform is the ACA of 2010 (Pub. L. 111-148), which was passed on March 23, 2010. This law is referred to by many names. In addition to its full title, it is also referred to as the Affordable Care Act, Obamacare, and as the abbreviations PPACA and ACA. General terms such as health care reform and health reform may also refer to the ACA. While portions of the law took place immediately, some significant portions began to take effect in 2014 and later. In summary, the ACA requires that most people in the United States have health insurance, using the methods of an individual mandate, employer requirements, and expansion of Medicaid. The ACA also includes rules for health care exchanges, requirements for health insurance plans, changes to Medicare and Medicaid services, and requirements regarding prevention and wellness services. The ACA primarily addresses the problem of access to health care, although some provisions also address cost and quality. The law impacts who receives coverage, what coverage is provided, and how services are provided.

One major issue that the ACA was intended to address was the high number of people in the United States who did not have health insurance. In 2012, 17.7% of people in the United States younger than 65 years of age were uninsured (Kaiser Commission on Medicaid and the Uninsured, 2013). Of those who had health insurance, 55.7% had employer-based insurance, 20.8% had Medicaid, and 5.8% had private nongroup insurance. Of those who did not have health insurance, 39% made less than the federal poverty level ($11,170 for an individual and $23,050 for a family of 4), and 10% made more than 400% of the federal poverty level ($44,680 for an individual and $92,200 for a family of 4; Kaiser Commission on Medicaid and the Uninsured, 2013). Lack of insurance restricts individuals' access to health services, including occupational therapy. In 2011, 26% of people without health insurance went without care, compared with 4% of those with health insurance (Askin & Moore, 2012). Studies have shown that people without health insurance experience health outcomes that are different from those with health insurance (Askin & Moore, 2012). Compared with those with health insurance, people without health insurance are diagnosed at later stages of disease, are more likely to be hospitalized, are less likely to receive diagnostic and therapeutic services in the hospital, are twice as likely to report being in fair or poor health, have more chronic medical conditions, and die earlier. When uninsured adults turned 65 years of age and started to receive Medicare, their overall health improved. These health outcomes may impact whether a person reaches a stage that requires occupational therapy and may impact the frequency of some chronic conditions that might be treated by occupational therapy.

Several components of the ACA are meant to address access to care, including the individual mandate, employer requirements, and Medicaid expansion. Under the individual mandate, the ACA requires that all U.S. citizens and legal residents have qualifying health coverage, with some exceptions. This mandate is enforced through tax penalties. Individuals without qualifying health coverage will receive a penalty, increasing in amount from 2014 to 2016. This mandate is supported through subsidies in the form of tax credits to help individuals afford health insurance. In addition, no one can be denied coverage due to a preexisting condition; rating variation can only be based on age, geographic area, family composition, and tobacco use. Young adults are also able to stay on their parents' insurance until the age of 26. Individuals who are exempted are the following: those experiencing financial hardship; those claiming a religious objection; American Indians; those who have been without coverage for less than 3 months; undocumented immigrants; those who are incarcerated; those having incomes for which the lowest-cost plan available exceeds 8%; and those with incomes below the tax filing threshold.

Employer-based insurance requirements are also meant to increase the number of people with health insurance. These requirements state that employers with more than 50 full-time employees will be required to pay a penalty if they do not offer affordable health insurance coverage. Employees may opt out of their employer-based plan. An employer with fewer than 50 full-time employees will not receive a penalty for not offering affordable coverage and may receive a tax credit if offering health insurance to employees (Kaiser Commission on Medicaid and the Uninsured, 2013).

The original form of the ACA included a requirement for the expansion of Medicaid to all non–Medicare-eligible individuals younger than 65 years age, with incomes up to 133% of the federal poverty level. As an example of who this would cover, in 2013, 133% of the federal poverty level was $15,281 for an individual and $31,322 for a family of four (Federal Register, 2013). A Supreme Court decision in 2012 limited the ability of the federal government to enforce this expansion, leaving the decision of Medicaid expansion up to each individual state. If a state decides to expand Medicaid, the federal government will pay for the additional coverage initially but will then phase out its financial support so that eventually the state will cover the additional cost. As of March 2015, 28 states and the District of Columbia have chosen to expand coverage. These states are Arizona, Arkansas, California, Colorado, Connecticut, Delaware, Hawaii, Illinois, Indiana, Iowa, Kentucky, Maryland, Massachusetts, Michigan, Minnesota, Nevada, New Hampshire, New Jersey, New Mexico, New York, North Dakota, Ohio, Oregon, Pennsylvania, Rhode Island, Vermont, Washington, and West Virginia. Although the expansion of Medicaid will result in many more people with health insurance, many Americans will remain uninsured. In states that do not expand Medicaid, a coverage gap will occur consisting of those who are not eligible for Medicaid and who are exempt from the individual mandate due to financial hardship or because they cannot find a plan that is less than 8% of their income and will likely remain uninsured. In addition, some individuals may choose to pay the tax penalty instead of buying insurance.

Although the ACA is primarily intended to address access to health care, it also aims to address the quality of care. Health reform addressing quality is challenging because the term *quality* is more difficult to define and measure than cost or access. Quality may be defined as care that is safe, effective, efficient, timely, equitable, or client centered. Often, quality is measured by the degree to which services increase desired outcomes and are consistent with current professional knowledge (Askin & Moore, 2012). Quality of care can be affected by administrative and systemic causes, as well as by clinician or client behavior. For example, some factors that influence quality of care include underuse of services when clients do not receive treatments that have shown to be effective, overuse of services when clients receive unnecessary treatment, and misuse of services such as hospital-acquired infections or falls that occur in inpatient settings (Askin & Moore, 2012).

To address quality of health care, the ACA establishes 10 categories of benefits that health insurance companies must cover. These minimum requirements, known as the essential benefits package, include the following:

1. Ambulatory patient services

2. Emergency services

3. Hospitalization

4. Maternity and newborn care

5. Mental health and substance use disorder services, including behavioral health treatment

6. Prescription drugs

7. Rehabilitative and habilitative services and devices

8. Laboratory services

9. Prevention and wellness services and chronic disease management

10. Pediatric services, including oral and vision care

Some of these requirements may have a direct impact on the practice of occupational therapy, especially in the areas of mental and behavioral health, rehabilitation and habilitation, outpatient and inpatient care, and wellness and chronic disease management (Braveman & Metzler, 2012).

The requirements for mental and behavioral health coverage state that coverage must be generally comparable to coverage for medical and surgical care. This requirement fulfills the previously passed requirements of the Mental Health Parity and Addiction Equity Act of 2008. For example, plans cannot set higher deductibles or charge higher copayments for mental health visits than for medical visits. Plans also cannot set more restrictive limits on the number of visits for mental health and cannot make getting prior approval for mental health treatment more difficult than for admission to an acute care hospital. Health plans must cover preventative services such as depression screening and behavioral assessments at no cost. Furthermore, preexisting mental illnesses cannot cause a person to be denied coverage. These requirements may allow people with mental health needs greater access to mental health care, and there is potential for occupational therapy practitioners to become more involved in such services.

Requirements regarding rehabilitative and habilitative services and devices will likely have a significant impact on the practice of occupational therapy. The inclusion of habilitative services and devices was a direct result of advocacy from the American Occupational Therapy Association (AOTA) and ensures that occupational therapy specifically for habilitation and rehabilitation, beyond the broad categories of hospital or outpatient services, is covered (Metzler, Tomlinson, Nanof, & Hitchon, 2012). The National Association of Insurance Commissioners (NAIC) created a glossary of terms in the essential health benefits to inform consumers and provide recommendations to federal agencies for providing coverage. Both habilitation and rehabilitation services are defined in the NAIC glossary. The AOTA advocated to the NAIC to specifically mention occupational therapy in both definitions:

> *Habilitation services:* Health care services that help a person keep, learn, or improve skills and functioning for daily living are habilitation services. Examples include therapy for a child who is not walking or talking at the expected age. These services may include physical and occupational therapy, speech–language pathology services, and other services for people with disabilities in a variety of inpatient and/or outpatient settings.
>
> *Rehabilitation services:* Rehabilitation services are health care services that help a person keep, regain, or improve skills and functioning for daily living that have been

lost or impaired because a person was sick, hurt, or disabled. These services may include physical and occupational therapy, speech–language pathology, and psychiatric rehabilitation services in a variety of inpatient and/or outpatient settings (NAIC, 2011, pp. 2-3).

While rehabilitative services help people regain skills they previously had, habilitative services help people learn or maintain functional skills that they did not previously have. Before the ACA, many insurance plans did not cover habilitative services because they claimed that learning a skill for the first time was educational and not medical. Despite the recommendations from the NAIC, states and insurance companies are able to make specific definitions of habilitative and rehabilitative services. If a state does not define habilitative services, the U.S. Department of Health and Human Services may allow insurance plans to use their own definitions, which may or may not include occupational therapy. Brown (2014) argues that to ensure that occupational therapy is included in these services, occupational therapy practitioners need to continue to be involved in the process of defining habilitative coverage.

The prevention services covered in the essential benefits package free of cost include blood pressure screening, cholesterol screening, depression screening, diabetes (type 2) screening, obesity screening and counseling, and vaccines. The ACA also establishes the National Prevention, Health Promotion, and Public Health Council, which is a group of 20 federal departments, agencies, and offices that coordinate federal prevention, wellness, and public health activities. This council includes representatives of the areas of housing, transportation, education, environment, and defense. Wellness services covered by the essential benefits package may include smoking cessation, weight management, stress management, physical fitness, nutrition, health disease prevention, healthy lifestyle support, and diabetes prevention. Employers can offer incentive-based wellness programs, and employees' insurance costs can be linked to their participation in such programs.

Despite these minimum requirements in the ACA, coverage may vary from state to state because the act does not define the scope and nature of coverage under these categories and does not address other issues that may arise when implementing these requirements (Metzler et al., 2012). Therefore, the role of occupational therapy in these requirements may be different in different states. States are able to choose a benchmark (a baseline of coverage) from existing health plans that qualify under the federal law. Although occupational therapy is covered in most plans that states can choose from for a benchmark, it is possible that there may be some cases in which occupational therapy is not covered by the benchmark plan (Metzler et al., 2012). Furthermore, if a benchmark plan does not include coverage of all the essential health benefit categories, qualified plans must adequately cover each category, creating potential gaps in coverage. New opportunities for occupational therapy may arise to fill these potential gaps (Metzler et al., 2012).

To address both quality and cost, the ACA emphasizes the importance of research and introduces new programs to find effective and efficient treatments. Several programs to address research may be relevant to occupational therapy practice. The Patient-Centered Outcomes Research Institute (PCORI) compares the effectiveness of medical treatments. The Supporting New Ideas in the Private Market program includes the research of new medical technology. To help people afford long-term care, the ACA has established the program Community Living Assistance Services and Supports (CLASS), which is a national, voluntary insurance program for long-term care. It provides a cash benefit to individuals with functional limitations so that they can purchase non-medical services and supports necessary to remain in community residence. Individuals qualify to receive the benefit when they need help with certain activities of daily living. The benefit can be used to maintain independence in the home or in the community through the use of home health services or adult daycare. The benefit may also be used to offset costs associated with assisted living and nursing home care.

Telehealth

Another part of the ACA that will likely impact the practice of occupational therapy is the act's mention of telehealth, a means of service that some occupational therapy practitioners already practice. The ACA mentions telehealth by name and makes reference to providing services through "telephonic or web-based intervention" (Patient Protection and Affordable Care Act, 2010, p. 33). Telehealth services can be used to address access, cost, or quality of care. Telehealth is referred to as a service means for wellness and prevention programs and for coordinated care for Medicare, Medicaid, and Accountable Care Organizations. Telehealth is permitted to be used in some situations that require a "face-to-face encounter," such as when physicians prescribe home health or review medications. Telehealth is also referred to as a method to improve the quality of services available to underserved populations and to be used in the expansion of community-based collaborative care networks. It may be possible for occupational therapists to become involved in some of these opportunities. Cason (2012) mentions several potential opportunities for occupational therapy practitioners. Practitioners can use telehealth to become involved in the areas of prevention and wellness, coordinated care, pediatric services, productive aging, mental health, rehabilitation, community participation, and work and industry.

Health Insurance Marketplace

To address the cost of health care, the ACA establishes health care exchanges, also known as the Health Insurance Marketplace. The exchanges allow individuals to determine the actual costs of plans and to compare policies based on price and coverage. The exchanges also create risk pools so that the total amounts the insurers pay are balanced between people with more expensive health needs and people with less expensive health needs. Insurance companies must meet all the minimum requirements of the essential benefits package to be allowed into the exchanges.

Accountable Care Organizations

To address cost in Medicare, the ACA introduces several new models of care. One new model, Accountable Care Organizations (ACOs), is an integrated network of providers including hospitals, outpatient clinics, primary care centers, community clinics, inpatient rehabilitation facilities, and private practitioners. Within the ACO, providers agree to work together to improve individual and population health, to coordinate care, and to share accountability for quality, costs, and health outcomes of patients. To qualify as an ACO, the network of providers must accept responsibility for at least 5,000 clients, establish a governing body that includes patients and providers, develop a plan for self-assessment and reporting of care, take responsibility for each client's entire continuum of care, and agree to participate for at least 3 years. ACOs are financially rewarded for saving costs, and providers can share in saving if they also meet certain quality standards. In this way, ACOs may address the rising health care costs, such as those caused by duplication of services and readmissions. The role of occupational therapy practitioners in ACOs is still being defined, but this may provide additional opportunities for the practice of occupational therapy (Lamb & Metzler, 2014).

Medical Home Model

Another similar model being tried out in Medicare is the Medical Home Model. Unlike ACOs, this model is led by personal physicians. Medical Home Models coordinate care from several different providers. The ACA is also addressing cost in Medicare through bundled payments, lump sums that Medicare will provide for a course of treatment of a specific disease or condition, rather than fee-for-service payments. The lump sum will cover hospital care, rehospitalization, post-acute care, physician services, and other services, including occupational therapy. Bundled payments are meant to reduce overall costs, focus responsibility, and prevent acute care services from shifting costs to post-acute care providers.

The ACA has already impacted health care in the United States, and changes will continue to occur as the final pieces take effect, as challenges are decided in the courts, and as states make new decisions. The ACA will continue to shape the experiences of individuals by impacting who will have access to insurance and what specific coverage and benefits will be available. Additional contexts will impact clients and practitioners, such as how clearly changes are communicated by the media, insurance companies, and health care providers, and access to technology. The ACA will continue to shape the demand for occupational therapy services and the ways in which these services are provided. Since the ACA provides incentives to provide high-quality care in an efficient manner, occupational therapy practitioners may have an opportunity to demonstrate how the profession's unique focus on evidence-based practice, client-centered care, and validated assessments can add value to provider networks and programs (Fisher & Friesema, 2013).

Individuals With Disabilities Education Act

The history of IDEA can also be traced to the Social Security Act of 1935, which included a section that provided funding to states to create Crippled Children Services. Occupational therapists began practicing in educational settings at this time, often in segregated settings working with children with orthopedic and neurological impairments (Swinth, 2014). In 1975, the Education for All Handicapped Children Act (EHA) was passed to ensure that all children ages 6 through 21 years receive a free and equal education in the least restrictive environment. The EHA also required schools to create Individualized Education Programs (IEPs) for children with disabilities (Dunn, 1988). Under this act, occupational therapy was identified as a related service available to students. The EHA was amended in 1986 to include services for children aged 3 to 5 years and to provide incentives for states to provide early intervention to younger children.

The EHA was expanded and renamed in 1990 with the passing of the IDEA, which placed a greater emphasis on the access of students with disabilities to education that is equal to that of their peers. The IDEA provides guidelines and protections to ensure that children with disabilities have access to free and appropriated public education (Hammel, Charlton, Jones, Kramer, & Wilson, 2014). Under this act, the federal government provides funds to states and local education agencies to support education for children with disabilities. The IDEA was further revised in 1997 and again in 2004. These revisions added the services of assistive technology, early intervention for age birth to 3 years, transitional services beginning at 14 years, and programs for students with emotional disturbances (Swinth, 2014). Under the IDEA, occupational therapy is identified as a related service for eligible children who require assistance to benefit from special education. Occupational therapy is also identified as a primary service for children from birth through age 2 years who are eligible to receive early intervention services (Swinth, Chandler, Hanft, Jackson, & Shepherd, 2003). In a school setting, occupational therapy intervention must help the student achieve educational goals related to supporting the student's performance within the educational environment. In this way, the IDEA has shaped the practice of occupational therapy. The IDEA demonstrates one way that legislation can have a significant impact on the field of occupational therapy. After the passing of the IDEA, education and early intervention became the areas with the most occupational therapy practitioners (Christiansen & Haertl, 2014).

Americans With Disabilities Act

The first federal legislation to prohibit discrimination against people with disabilities was the Rehabilitation Act of 1973, Section 504 (Eichhorn, 1998). The Rehabilitation Act of 1973 applies only to programs of the federal government, programs that receive federal financial assistance, and programs that contract with the federal government. In 1990, the ADA was passed to extend civil rights to people with disabilities in all areas of society. The ADA sought to provide protection against discrimination for people with disabilities that are similar to protections provided on the basis of race, color, sex, national origin, age, and religion. Under the ADA, individuals with disabilities have the right to equal access to opportunities to live, work, and play within society. The act provides equal opportunities in employment, state and local government services, public accommodations, commercial facilities, and transportation. The ADA was amended in 2008 to address the original act's narrow definition of "a person with a disability" and to place less emphasis on the need for individuals to prove the severity of an impairment in order to receive protection (Hammel et al., 2014).

The ADA impacts both the experiences of individuals whom occupational therapy practitioners may work with and the practice of occupational therapy. The act shapes the settings that occupational practitioners work in and what they might do in those settings. For example, practitioners may contribute to ensuring equal access by helping to develop reasonable accommodations, independent living skills, or compensatory strategies that minimize functional limitations (AOTA, 2000). The act can also guide practitioners in their roles as advocates with clients if practitioners are aware of what opportunities or services may be available for clients (Hammel et al., 2014).

CONCLUSION

Contexts of legislation, geography, and demographics can have a significant impact on occupational therapy practitioners and clients. Many clients, such as Ruth introduced at the beginning of the chapter, may need assistance in understanding how changes in legislation impact the health coverage they may receive. However, as occupational therapy practitioners, we must also be aware of how clients' experiences in interacting with systems of health care, education, and community services have been shaped by specific historical, political, and social contexts. Understanding these contexts can help practitioners ensure that they are providing the best care available to their clients. Furthermore, it may be possible to anticipate future changes in policies and advocate for a greater role of occupational therapy in additional services.

SUGGESTED WEBSITES

- Official federal government webpage: https://www.healthcare.gov/
- American Occupational Therapy Association site with updates about the ACA relevant to occupational therapy practitioners: http://www.aota.org/Advocacy-Policy/Health-Care-Reform.aspx
- The Kaiser Family Foundation, a non-profit organization that provides information on national health issues, including up-to-date information about health care reform: http://kff.org/health-reform/

REVIEW QUESTIONS

1. What three components of health care reform are said to be in an interdependent "iron triangle"?

   a. Medicare, Medicaid, and Social Security

   b. Cost, access, and quality

   c. Hospitals, physicians, and insurance companies

   d. Geography, demographics, and cost

2. Which program provides health insurance to individuals over the age of 65, individuals with disabilities, individuals with amyotrophic lateral sclerosis (ALS), and individuals in need of dialysis or a kidney transplant?

   a. Medicaid

   b. Social Security

   b. Medicare

   c. Americans with Disabilities Act (ADA)

3. Which program provides financial support to states to provide health insurance to individuals who qualify based on their income?

   a. Medicaid

   b. Social Security

   c. Medicare

   d. Patient Protection and ACA

4. The 1935 Social Security Act included precursors to all of the following programs except:

   a. Medicare

   b. Individuals with Disabilities Education Act (IDEA)

   c. Accountable Care Organizations (ACOs)

   d. Children's Health Insurance Program (CHIP)

5. In what year was Medicare passed?

   a. 1935

   b. 1965

   c. 1973

   d. 2010

6. Which is the largest payer of health care in the United States?

   a. Medicare

   b. Medicaid

   c. Blue Cross–Blue Shield

   d. Individuals with private, nongroup insurance

7. What group of individuals is not required to be covered under Medicaid?

   a. Children

   b. Parents with dependent children

   c. People with severe disabilities

   d. Adults older than 21 years of age

8. Which requirement of the ACA attempts to increase the number of Americans with health insurance?

   a. Minimum benefits package

   b. Accountable care organizations

   c. The individual mandate

   d. Medicare

9. Which of the following is not a minimum requirement for health insurance coverage under the ACA?

   a. Dental and vision care for individuals older than 65 years of age

   b. Mental health, substance use services, and behavioral health

   c. Rehabilitative and habilitative services

   d. Prevention and wellness services

10. Which act currently provides funds to support access of students with disabilities to education that is equal to that of their peers?

    a. EHA

    b. IDEA

    c. Medicaid

    d. ACA

REFERENCES

American Occupational Therapy Association. (2000). Occupational therapy and the Americans with Disabilities Act (ADA). *American Journal of Occupational Therapy, 54,* 622-625.

Askin, E., & Moore, N. (2012). *The health care handbook: A clear and concise guide to the United States health care system.* St. Louis: Washington University.

Braveman, B., & Metzler, C. A. (2012). Health care reform implementation and occupational therapy. *American Journal of Occupational Therapy, 66*(1), 11-14.

Brown, D. (2014). Health policy perspectives—habilitative services: An essential health benefit and an opportunity for occupational therapy practitioners and consumers. *American Journal of Occupational Therapy, 68,* 130–138.

Cason, J. (2012). Telehealth opportunities in occupational therapy through the Affordable Care Act. *American Journal of Occupational Therapy, 66*(2), 131-136.

Christiansen, C. H., & Haertl, K. (2014). A contextual history of occupational therapy. In B. A. B. Schell, G. Gillen, & M. F. Scaffa (Eds.), *Willard and Spackman's occupational therapy* (12th ed., pp. 9-34). Philadelphia: Lippincott Williams & Wilkins.

Cohen, W. J. (1983). The development of the Social Security Act of 1935: Reflections some fifty years later. *Minnesota Law Review, 68,* 379.

Dunn, W. (1988). Models of occupational therapy service provision in the school system. *American Journal of Occupational Therapy, 42*(11), 718-723.

Eichhorn, L. (1998). Major litigation activities regarding major life activities: The failure of the disability definition in the Americans with Disabilities Act of 1990. *North Carolina Law Review, 77,* 1405.

Federal Register, Vol. 78, No. 16, January 24, 2013. Retrieved from https://federalregister.gov/a/2013-01422

Fisher, G., & Friesema, J. (2013). Implications of the Affordable Care Act for occupational therapy practitioners providing services to Medicare recipients. *American Journal of Occupational Therapy, 67*(5), 502-506.

Freedman, M. K. (2012). Special education: Its ethical dilemmas, entitlement status, and suggested systemic reforms. *University of Chicago Law Review, 79*, 1-4.

Hammel, J., Charlton, J., Jones, R. A., Kramer, J. M., Wilson, T. (2014). Disability rights and advocacy. In B. A. B. Schell, G. Gillen, & M. F. Scaffa (Eds.), *Willard and Spackman's occupational therapy* (12th ed., pp. 1031-1050). Philadelphia: Lippincott Williams & Wilkins.

Kaiser Commission on Medicaid and the Uninsured. (2013). *The uninsured: A primer.* Retrieved from http://kff.org/uninsured/report/the-uninsured-a-primer-key-facts-about-health-insurance-on-the-eve-of-coverage-expansions/

Kronenfeld, J. J. (2011). *Medicare.* Santa Barbara, CA: Greenwood.

Lamb, A. J., & Metzler, C. A. (2014). Health policy perspectives—defining the value of occupational therapy: A health policy lens on research and practice. *American Journal of Occupational Therapy, 68*, 9–14. http://dx.doi.org/10.5014/ajot.2014.681001

Lohman, H. (2014). Payment for services in the United States. In B. A. B. Schell, G. Gillen, & M. F. Scaffa (Eds.), *Willard and Spackman's occupational therapy* (12th ed., pp. 1051-1067). Philadelphia: Lippincott Williams & Wilkins.

Mehta, N., & Jha S. (2012). The Patient Protection and Affordable Care Act in a nutshell. *Journal of the American College of Radiology, 9*(12), 877-880.

Metzler, C., Tomlinson, J., Nanof, T., & Hitchon, J. (2012). Health policy perspectives—what is essential in the essential health benefits? And will occupational therapy benefit? *American Journal of Occupational Therapy, 66*, 389–394. http://dx.doi.org/10.5014/ajot.2012.664001

National Association of Insurance Commissioners. (2011, July). Uniform glossary and summary of benefits and coverage, final submission. Retrieved from www.naic.org/documents/committees_b_consumer_information_ppaca_glossary.pdf

Parks, D. (2012). *Health care reform simplified: What professionals in medicine, government, insurance, and business need to know.* New York: Apress.

Patient Protection and Affordable Care Act, 42 U.S.C. § 18001 (2010). Retrieved from http://www.hhs.gov/healthcare/rights/law/patient-protection.pdf

Rothman, D. (2005). A century of failure: Health care reform in America. In P. Conrad (Ed.), *The sociology of health and illness: Critical perspectives* (7th ed., pp. 292-300). New York: Worth.

Swinth, Y.L. (2014). Education. In B. A. B. Schell, G. Gillen, & M. F. Scaffa (Eds.), *Willard and Spackman's occupational therapy* (12th ed., pp. 653-677). Philadelphia: Lippincott Williams & Wilkins.

Swinth, Y., Chandler, B., Hanft, B., Jackson, L., & Shepherd, J. (2003). *Personnel issues in school-based occupational therapy: Supply and demand, preparation, certification and licensure. COPSSE Document No. IB-1.* Gainesville, FL: University of Florida, Center on Personnel Studies in Special Education.

2

Leadership and Advocacy

Sarah McKinnon, MS, OTR/L

"Leadership is not simply a position, but rather a willingness to make a significant difference and have a lasting impact on those around you."

—Jeff Snodgrass (2011, p. 272)

ACOTE Standard explored in this chapter:

- B.6.4. Identify the role and responsibility of the practitioner to advocate for changes in service delivery policies, to effect changes in the system, and to recognize opportunities in emerging practice areas.

KEY VOCABULARY

Leadership: A practice of encouraging others to purposefully accomplish an outcome that will achieve the fullest potential of the individual, department, profession, or community.

Transactional leadership: A leadership style based on exchanges between a leader and a follower, in which followers are rewarded only after meeting specific goals or exceeding performance criteria.

Transformational leadership: A leadership style in which leaders create connections with followers, inspiring and motivating others to exceed an outcome beyond exchanges and rewards.

Emotional intelligence: The ability to perceive, access, generate, and regulate emotions to promote emotional and intellectual growth.

Self-awareness: The understanding of one's own emotions, strengths, weaknesses, needs, and drives.

Self-regulation: The ability to manage emotions, moods, and impulses and channel them in useful ways.

Jacobs K, ed.
Management and Administration for the OTA:
Leadership and Application Skills (pp 15-32).

Motivation: The ability to increase one's desire to achieve a goal or desired outcome.

Advocacy: The process of supporting a cause, such as an idea, policy, or activity, that can directly affect a person or group's well-being.

Health policy: A written statement that describes the intended course of an issue related to health.

Political action committee (PAC): A committee that provides funding to state and federal candidates who support a profession or industry and their initiatives through private donations from association members. AOTPAC is The American Occupational Therapy Political Action Committee, which is the PAC for American Occupational Therapy Association (AOTA) members.

The concept of leadership has been explored extensively over the past century, with recent examination of the influence of leadership in health care, specifically rehabilitation therapies. In fact, the significance of leadership development in occupational therapy practice has led to the incorporation of leadership development as part of the *AOTA Strategic Goals 2013–2017* (AOTA, 2013). The importance of leadership has become an essential tool for practitioners, as evidenced by the development of AOTA initiatives such as the Emerging Leaders Development Program and the Leadership Development Program for Managers. The topic of leadership has also emerged in occupational therapy assistant (OTA) education curricula to align with ACOTE standards.

The purpose of this chapter is to identify the role of leadership in occupational therapy practice and to identify the relationships in which occupational therapy practitioners and students can become leaders. Common leadership theories, effective leadership skills, and activities in various environments that foster leadership development will be explained. In addition, the power of advocacy, a component of leadership, is described, and the opportunities to be a powerful occupational therapy advocate are discussed.

LEADERSHIP

Leadership is the practice of encouraging others to purposefully accomplish an outcome that will achieve the fullest potential of the individual, department, profession, or community. Definitions of leadership may vary in different professions, but within occupational therapy, leadership is an action to motivate clients, families, colleagues, and fellow team members to produce goals for optimal participation, independence, and quality of life. Nowhere in this definition is the term "manager" used. All occupational therapy practitioners must be leaders, even if the job title does not include it.

LEADERSHIP STYLES IN HEALTH CARE

Leadership is a practice requiring action, and the delivery of effective leadership strategies can differ across departments, organizations, or sectors. A leadership strategy that may be effective for one occupational therapy department, setting, or practice area may not be effective for another. Strategies used within a small group, department, or professional organization may be similar, but because there is a variety of settings in which leadership occurs, it is important to understand the diverse leadership theories and the ideas on which leadership is based.

Transactional leadership is a style that is based on exchanges between a leader and a follower or colleague in which followers are rewarded only when meeting specific goals or exceeding performance criteria (Aarons, 2006). In this style, the leader identifies the role and designates necessary tasks to followers while providing positive and negative rewards based on performance. The transactional leadership style is often characterized by the use of rewards or the avoidance of penalties, while also monitoring the occurrence of mistakes (Snodgrass, 2011). An example of transactional

CASE STUDY

Jen had been an OTA for 5 years when she decided she was ready to contribute to her profession in a different way. Her experiences primarily working with adults increased her confidence to discuss the role of occupational therapy and communicate the value of occupational therapy interventions firsthand within her client populations.

While reviewing her professional goals, Jen decided that she wanted to pursue more opportunities related to federal advocacy. She had been a member of both AOTA and her state association for years but thought that she could involve herself more than just renewing her membership annually. Jen decided to make a goal to attend the next AOTA Hill Day.

Upon arrival at Capitol Hill on AOTA Hill Day, Jen was excited when she was oriented to ongoing legislation related to occupational therapy because she often felt the struggle to stay current with legislation at home. Throughout her day, Jen joined other OTs, OTAs, and students to meet with senators and House representatives from her state and congressional district. To speak with legislators and their staffs was an opportunity she could not be more passionate about.

Back at work, Jen spoke of her experiences during an informal lunch presentation. Jen was able to describe her positive experience and encourage her department to contact state and federal legislators to support legislation related to occupational therapy. She was also able to describe firsthand the role of AOTPAC and the importance of AOTA membership. Jen's experience eventually created a trickle-down effect on her colleagues, and three of them attended their state's Hill Day the following spring.

leadership in use may be to grant a monetary reward for meeting productivity or to cancel a program or deny a request if expectations are not met.

On the other hand, transformational leadership is a style in which leaders create connections with followers that inspires and motivates others to exceed an outcome beyond exchanges and rewards (Aarons, 2006). Leaders using a transformational style tend to have a greater influence on employee and colleague satisfaction by also targeting intrinsic motivators of people involved (Aarons, 2006; Snodgrass, 2011). Transformational leadership can also be characterized by a close supervision relationship—one that can be paralleled to the occupational therapist (OT) and OTA relationship, as well as the OTA and OTA-student relationship during fieldwork experiences.

As evidenced by the identified leadership styles, measurement of the success of leadership can be recognized subjectively or objectively. Most commonly in the rehabilitation field where relationships are valued at the client, team, and community levels, successful leadership is viewed subjectively; that is, with use of opinions or personal feelings to determine a common good. As members of a department or organization view a leader, characteristics of success are not necessarily due to numeric outcomes or objective data. Rather, personal opinions and subjective comments are often deemed as effectiveness of leaders. Therefore, it is important to understand not only the differences in leadership theories, but also the skills of a successful leader, regardless of job title, role, or setting.

CHARACTERISTICS OF A SUCCESSFUL LEADER

In a school, work, or community setting, it is possible to identify individuals in leadership roles who have failed, and others who have excelled. Why are some people better leaders than others? As introduced in the previous section, particular leadership styles can warrant different outcomes based on the tone and relationship of the leader and colleague. In addition, personal styles of superb leaders can also vary, as some leaders are quiet and analytical while others are loud and

Figure 2-1. Leadership skills of emotional intelligence.

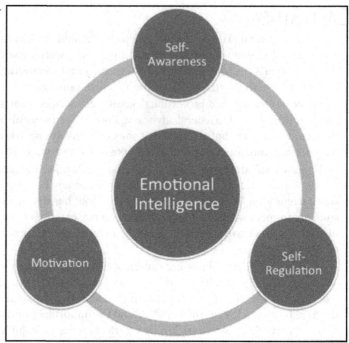

direct. Just as important, different situations call for different types of leadership. Leadership research over the past two decades has identified that although leaders can be different in many ways, the most effective leaders have a high degree of emotional intelligence (Goleman, 1998).

Emotional Intelligence

Emotional intelligence is the ability to perceive, access, generate, and regulate emotions to promote emotional and intellectual growth (Mayer & Salovey, 1997). The importance of emotional intelligence in people is supported by evidence-based research. For example, in a study where technical skills, intelligence quotient (IQ), and emotional intelligence were identified as the three primary groups of leadership characteristics, emotional intelligence proved to be twice as important as the other two (Goleman, 1998). Of course, IQ and technical skills are necessary characteristics of a skilled professional; however, without emotional intelligence, people may have the best training in the world but may lack necessary characteristics of a successful leader. What are specific skills of emotional intelligence and how can these skills be developed as an OTA? Self-awareness, self-regulation, and motivation are three skills of emotional intelligence that an occupational therapy practitioner can develop to become an excellent leader (Figure 2-1).

Self-Awareness

Self-awareness is a component of emotional intelligence in which an individual has a deep understanding of one's own emotions, strengths, weaknesses, needs, and drives. People with high self-awareness often know their effect on others and recognize how feelings affect themselves and the people with whom they work. In addition, individuals with high self-awareness have a good sense of goals and values, often finding work to be energizing. For example, an OTA with high self-awareness would recognize strengths and areas of improvement in clinical practice or communication, for example, and implement strategies to improve these skills while working with clients and fellow colleagues. In the case study, Jen is aware of her increasing confidence and identifies participation in advocacy as an area of improvement for professional development. Self-awareness can also be highlighted when writing professional goals as a student or as a clinician. In addition, this skill may be influential in an interview: "Tell me about your biggest area of improvement, and what you are doing to improve it." Self-aware candidates will be frank in admitting strengths and areas of improvement, but also are able to confidently explain strategies for self-improvement.

Self-Regulation

Self-regulation is the ability to manage emotions, moods, and impulses and channel these feelings in useful ways. People with high self-regulation typically exhibit compassionate and professional behaviors. For example, an individual who is in control of his or her feelings or impulses is often reasonable and can create an environment in the classroom or office with trust and fairness. People do not want to be yelled at, be judged openly, or be part of an unprofessional environment. Poor self-regulation and frustration can be viewed as complaining or aggressive and can create a negative work environment. Low morale or termination can be a result of impulsive behavior and poor self-regulation.

Self-regulation incorporates professional behaviors that are developed early in one's career in clinical practice. In the ever-changing health care environment, it is also important to develop self-regulation to adapt for change. External stressors may continue to affect the occupational therapy practice, influencing reimbursement, billing, and coding of procedures (see Chapter 4). In addition, changes in department budgets may also affect work-life balance, such as employee benefits or paid time off. It is important to regulate emotions from potentially stressful situations and continue to demonstrate professional behavior in the workplace. Although changes within the health care system or individual workplace resources may elicit testing of self-regulation, one must continue to provide excellent client-centered practice. In the case study, Jen described meeting with elected officials to discuss the importance of occupational therapy services in optimal client outcomes. In these conversations, Jen likely had to self-regulate her emotions in order to present her passion for occupational therapy in a professional manner.

Motivation

Motivation is the ability to increase one's desire to achieve a goal or desired outcome. Researchers have studied a variety of motivational theories that explain the desire for an individual to participate in activities, particularly work. Whereas some people are motivated by extrinsic factors, such as salaries and monetary benefits, many other people are motivated by intrinsic factors, such as self-worth, morals, and goals to seek out challenges. Often, people motivated by intrinsic factors and the desire to achieve for the sake of achievement have a trickle-down effect on fellow colleagues. For example, an OTA choosing to publish a case study in AOTA's *OT Practice* publication for the purpose of showcasing client-based and evidence-based intervention achievements may motivate a fellow colleague to also publish or present a case study at work. Even Jen's informal presentation to her colleagues about AOTA Hill Day inspired some of her coworkers to advocate for the OT profession and participate in state advocacy events.

It is not difficult to acknowledge why motivation can translate into effective leadership. If an individual or leader sets lofty, but achievable, individual goals, one can assume that this individual will do the same for a department or professional organization or in a community setting. Motivation by intrinsic versus extrinsic factors is common for occupational therapy practitioners. A prospective OTA student who pursues an education in occupational therapy likely is not motivated solely by extrinsic rewards, such as monetary compensation. It is reasonable to assume that individuals in rehabilitation fields choose to enter the field because of many intrinsic motivators, one of which is to improve the lives of other people. How motivating is that? During patient care interactions, OTAs are all leaders because they must motivate patients to achieve their highest potential for optimal participation in activities.

Figure 2-2. Primary relationships for OT leadership.

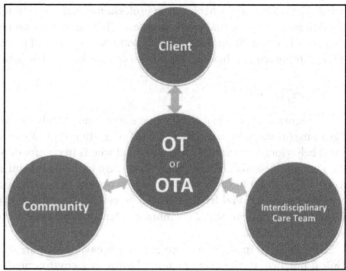

Summary

Self-awareness, self-regulation, and motivation are just three characteristics of successful and effective leaders that contribute to high emotional intelligence. It is important to note that these skills can be learned and continuously developed through one's life experiences, including OTA education and OTA practice. Consequently, having more years of work experience may contribute to the ability to develop these skills; however, new practitioners can be very strong in these leadership skills early in their practice and be able to lead others in a variety of environments, regardless of years of experience. Although emotional intelligence was identified in research as a strong component of successful leadership, IQ and clinical skills are also important ingredients for strong leadership and cannot be completely ignored when discussing successful leaders (Goleman, 1998). Emotional intelligence was once nice to have in a leader, but now it is a necessary trait. These skills must be continued to be self-evaluated by occupational therapy practitioners on a continual basis.

RELATIONSHIPS IN WHICH AN OCCUPATIONAL THERAPY PRACTITIONER CAN BE A LEADER

OTs and OTAs are constantly seeking ways to become leaders within the work and community environments. At first glance, opportunities may be scarce, as there are overwhelmingly more clinical staff positions than managerial positions. It is important to note, however, that nowhere does the leadership definition in this chapter exclusively use the term "manager." Consequently, there are opportunities to be a leader in occupational therapy without being in an authoritative role.

This section identifies the four primary relationships that an OT, OTA, and occupational therapy student are a part of that can elicit leadership opportunities. These relationships are based on clinical experiences and evidence. They include the following (Figure 2-2):

- The relationship between the occupational therapy practitioner and self
- The relationship between the occupational therapy practitioner and the client
- The relationship between the occupational therapy practitioner and the interdisciplinary team
- The relationship between the occupational therapy practitioner and the community

Relationship Between the Occupational Therapy Practitioner and Self

The center of this model is the relationship an occupational therapy practitioner has with him or herself. An individual must understand his or her strengths, weaknesses, goals, and motivators to be a leader. Having strong self-awareness, a component of emotional intelligence, is essential to this relationship as an OTA. Self-reflection and knowledge of one's strengths and weaknesses can increase leadership potential. In the case study, Jen demonstrated this relationship by self-reflecting and establishing goals related to advocacy.

In addition, people with emotional intelligence are more likely to outperform and have higher department satisfaction as leaders than individuals without emotional intelligence (Mayer & Salovey, 1997). The process of professional development begins early in the career of an OTA, starting with self-reflection during school. Development of these skills in professional goal writing, participation in the leadership development courses, or administration of self-assessment tools can improve the relationship an OTA has with himself or herself. This relationship will affect, but enhance, the remaining three relationships.

Relationship Between the Occupational Therapy Practitioner and the Client

The second relationship imperative in practice and that can also elicit leadership development is the one an occupational therapy practitioner has with the client. The AOTA's 2014 *Occupational Therapy Practice Framework* defines the client as "person, groups, or populations" (p. S2). This relationship with the client occurs in everyday practice and can be seen as the most important of these four relationships, given people's reasons for being OTAs in the first place—to make an impact on the quality of life and independence of an individual, group, or population. The relationship with the client occurs with one-to-one or group interventions and is present in the hospital, home health, and community settings, among other contexts.

The relationship between the OTA and client is also evident through the term *client-centered practice*, which is paramount to the scope of occupational therapy. This relationship incorporates respect for and partnership with clients as active participants in the therapy process. An OTA has the ability to be very creative in this relationship and stand out in numerous ways, whether providing a unique service delivery of an intervention, gaining information in a unique way (if a client is unable to communicate, for example), or incorporating evidence-based practice. An OTA can be a leader in this relationship by visibly incorporating evidence-based practice through the use of AOTA systematic reviews or critically appraised topics to the department. Verbalizing the use of evidence-based practice in the moment with a client can also build trust and enhance this relationship. An OTA can also be a leader by connecting families to support groups, by networking support systems, or by creating written handouts that can be used for groups and populations. Obtaining AOTA board or specialty certification is another example of how the OTA can strengthen skills for this relationship and be a leader in the field. Participation in leadership activities will enhance personal and professional development but is also recognized for necessary credits for recertification by the National Board for Certification in Occupational Therapy (NBCOT) every 3 years (see Figure 2-3).

Relationship Between the Occupational Therapy Practitioner and the Interdisciplinary Care Team

The relationship between the occupational therapy practitioner and the interdisciplinary care team is essential for optimal communication and collaboration for excellent patient care. The

NBCOT® Professional Development Units (PDU) Activities Chart

PDU ID#	Professional Development Activity	PDU Value	Max units allowed per 3 year cycle	Verification Documentation
PROFESSIONAL SERVICE				
1	Assessing professional skills using the NBCOT Self-Assessment tool(s) (available online at www.nbcot.org) or similar professional skills assessment tool, (e.g., AOTA or employer-based professional development tool).	1 unit per tool	7 units (for completing a maximum of 7 NBCOT self-assessment tools)	Print off score report from NBCOT online self-assessment; or provide copy of completed tool from other providers
2	Developing a Professional Development Plan based on the results of a professional skills assessment.	1 unit	1 unit	Use results of self-assessment tool(s) (see above) to develop goals relating to competence/skills.
3	Volunteering for an organization, population, or individual that adds to the overall development of one's practice roles.	5 hours = 1 unit	18 units	Verification of hours via letter from organization and a report describing the hours and outcomes of volunteer service. Volunteer Service form is available online at www.nbcot.org.
4	Peer review of a professional manuscript or textbook.	2 hours = 1 unit	18 units	Letter from publishing organization.
5	Mentoring an OT colleague or other professional to improve skills of the protégé, including role as a disciplinary monitor (mentor must be currently certified with NBCOT).	2 hours = 1 unit	18 units	Goals, objectives, and analysis of mentee performance (see NBCOT Mentoring form, at www.nbcot.org).
ATTENDING WORKSHOPS/COURSES/INDEPENDENT LEARNING				
6	Attending employer-provided, workplace continuing education (this may include CPR training). *Does not include new staff orientation and/or annual mandatory workplace trainings e.g. annual policy review and corporate compliance. The same workshop may be claimed one-time only for PDU.*	1 hour = 1 unit	36 units	A certificate of attendance or letter from sponsor/employer verifying contact hours or CEU, dates, event title, attendee name and workshop agenda (if available).
7	Attending workshops, seminars, lectures, professional conferences approved by one of the following (same workshop may be claimed one-time only for PDU): 1) Regionally accredited college or university; 2) State regulatory board for licensure renewal; 3) Continuing education providers (e.g., state associations, continuing education companies); 4) Third-party entity.	1 hour = 1 unit	36 units	A certificate of attendance or letter from sponsor/employer verifying contact hours or CEU, dates, event title, attendee name and workshop agenda (if available)
8	Successfully completing education (e.g., workshops, seminars, lectures, online courses or conferences) with an assessment component at the end of the program (e.g., scored test, project, paper) provided by: • AOTA • AOTA approved providers • IACET authorized providers • Regionally accredited colleges or universities	1 hour = 1.25 units	36 units	Certificate of attendance or letter from education provider (AOTA, AOTA approved providers, IACET authorized providers or regionally accredited college or university) verifying dates, event title, attendee name, agenda, and successful completion of assessment component at the end of the program (e.g., scored test, project, paper).
9	Reading peer-reviewed, role-related professional journal article and/or textbook chapter, and writing a report describing the implications for improving skills in one's specific role (Cannot claim for PDU purposes if textbook is required reading for academic coursework/audited course).	2 articles or 2 chapters = 1 unit	36 units	Annotated bibliography AND a report with analysis of how articles have assisted with improving skills in one's role (see Journal/Text Book Reading form, at www.nbcot.org).
10	Successfully completing academic coursework. Course must relate to practice area.	1 credit hour/ per semester = 10 units	36 units	Official transcript from accredited college/university with registrar's seal. This should be placed in a sealed envelope, with 'RENEWAL' noted on the exterior. Send this envelope **with** your renewal application. DO NOT SEND TRANSCRIPT SEPARATELY.
11	Independent learning *with* assessment component (e.g., online courses, CE articles, self-study series, etc.).	1 hour = 1 unit	36 units	Certificate of completion verifying contact hours or CEU.
12	Independent learning *without* assessment component (e.g., audited coursework, multimedia courses, etc.).	2 hours = 1 unit	18 units	Summary report of learning with notation of hours spent.
13	Receiving mentoring from a currently certified occupational therapy practitioner or other professional in good standing to improve the skills of the protégé.	2 hours = 1 unit	18 units	Goals and objectives established in collaboration with the mentor and self-analysis of performance (see NBCOT Mentoring form, at www.nbcot.org).
14	Participating in professional study group/online study group designed to advance knowledge through active participation.	2 hours = 1 unit	18 units	Group attendance records verifying time spent, study group goals, and analysis of goal attainment and learning (see Study Group Report form, at www.nbcot.org).

Figure 2-3. Sample chart audit. (Reprinted with permission from NBCOT, http://www.nbcot.org/assets/candidate-pdfs/practitioner-pdfs/pdu_chart.pdf.) *(continued)*

PDU ID#	Professional Development Activity	PDU Value	Max units allowed per 3 year cycle	Verification Documentation
PRESENTING				
15	Primary or co-presenter making a professional presentation at state, national or international workshop, seminar, or conference (one-time presentation per topic; time spent on preparation cannot be included).	1 hour = 2 units	36 units	Copy of presentation OR copy of program listing. Presenter name and times (or length of session) and title of presentation must be indicated on documentation.
16	Primary or co-presenter making a poster presentation for state, national, or international workshop, seminar, or conference (one-time presentation per topic; time spent on preparation cannot be included).	2 units per poster	18 units	Copy of presentation OR program listing. Presenter name and times (or length of session) and title of presentation must be indicated on documentation.
17	Serving as adjunct faculty, teaching practice area-related academic course per semester (must not be one's primary role; one-time per course title; time spent on preparation cannot be included) Note: For a one-time lecture, use PDU ID#18.	1 credit hour = 6 units	36 units	Letter of verification from school that includes dates, lecture/course title, length of session and course/lecture goals and objectives or copy of course syllabi.
18	Primary or co-presenter providing professional in-service training, instruction, or guest lecturer for occupational therapists, occupational therapy assistants, or related professionals (one-time presentation per topic; time spent on preparation cannot be included).	1 hour = 1 unit	18 units	Copy of attendance record and outline of presentation or letter from supervisor on letterhead verifying: presenter's name, date/time/length of presentation.
19	Primary or co-presenter providing presentation for local organization/ association/ group on practice area-related topic; e.g., energy conservation, back care and prevention of injury (one-time presentation per topic; time spent on preparation cannot be included).	1 hour = 1 unit	18 units	Copy of presentation or program listing that includes: presenter's name; date, time, and location of presentation; and contact person for organization.
FIELDWORK SUPERVISION				
20	Level I fieldwork direct supervision (must not be one's primary role).	1 unit per student	18 units	Letter of verification or certificate from school including dates of fieldwork and name of fieldwork student.
21	Level II fieldwork direct supervision (must not be one's primary role).	1 unit per 1 week of supervision per student supervised	18 units	Letter of verification or certificate from school that includes the dates of fieldwork. DO NOT submit student evaluation form as verification. Co-supervision is acceptable; record dates and times when acting as primary student supervisor. Supervision of more than one student at a time is acceptable; record dates and times of supervision provided to each student. Apply appropriate PDU number based on time spent supervising.
22	Entry-level or post-doctoral advanced fieldwork direct supervision (must not be one's primary role).	1 unit per 1 week of supervision per student supervised	18 units	Letter of verification or certificate from school that includes the dates of fieldwork. DO NOT submit student evaluation form as verification. Co-supervision is acceptable; record dates and times when acting as primary student supervisor. Supervision of more than one student at a time is acceptable; record dates and times of supervision provided to each student. Apply appropriate PDU number based on time spent supervising.
PUBLISHING				
23	Primary or co-author of practice-area related article in non-peer-reviewed professional publication (e.g., *OT Practice, SIS Quarterly, Advance*).	1 article = 5 units	36 units	Copy of published article.
24	Primary or co-author of practice-area related article in peer-reviewed professional publication (e.g., journal, book chapter, or research paper.)	1 article = 10 units	36 units	Copy of published article.
25	Primary or co-author of practice-area related article in lay publication (e.g., community newspaper or newsletter).	1 article = 2 units	36 units	Copy of published article.
26	Primary or co-author of chapter in practice-area related professional textbook.	1 chapter = 10 units	36 units	Copy of published chapter OR letter from editor.
27	Primary or co-primary investigator in extensive scholarly research activities or outcome studies, or externally funded service/training projects associated with grants or post-graduate studies.	10 units per study	18 units	Grant funding number OR abstract/executive summary OR copy of the completed research/study that indicates certificant as primary/co-primary investigator.
28	Developing instructional materials—training manuals, multimedia, or software programs—that advance the professional skills of others (not for proprietary use; must not be part of one's primary role)	5 units	18 units	Program description (Note: Media and software materials may be requested by NBCOT).

ID 51 rev11/25/2013

Figure 2-3 (continued). Sample chart audit.

interdisciplinary care team includes members of the team who are assuming responsibility of a client's care. Members of this team include physicians, nurses, case managers, occupational therapy practitioners, physical therapy practitioners, speech pathologists, social workers, and more. This relationship is visible in the clinical setting, especially where multiple disciplines provide care in one building. In the acute care environment, there have been more initiatives for team rounds, something that is prevalent in the inpatient rehabilitation facility setting. This relationship is also beginning to blossom in the outpatient and community settings in the area of primary care and chronic illness, two emerging practices of occupational therapy.

Research suggests that multidisciplinary teams are more effective than control groups for increasing patient outcomes and satisfaction and decreasing lengths of stay for certain populations (Hand, Law, & McCool, 2011). The relationship between an occupational therapy practitioner and the members of the interdisciplinary team is important not only for advocacy for occupational therapy, but also for the care and outcomes of clients. Opportunities to strengthen this relationship and lead within the occupational therapy field can be presented in many creative ways. Entry-level OTAs may be surprised to know that many disciplines do not know what occupational therapy practitioners do. Interdisciplinary rounds are a great way to increase awareness of the role of occupational therapy and strengthen the morale of the care team, while providing the best patient care. Although these rounds may be attended by the primary OT, it is important to recognize the members of the interdisciplinary team and be as present as possible to advocate for the client and for occupational therapy.

An occupational therapy practitioner can also strengthen the relationship with the interprofessional care team through writing and presenting. Is there an e-mail "blast" or department newsletter published in the hospital that could showcase the department? Is there a forum to present the role of occupational therapy and interventional outcomes at an in-service? Being present will increase the importance of occupational therapy in the eyes of those who are unfamiliar with the profession.

Relationship Between the Occupational Therapy Practitioner and the Community

The final relationship identified for leadership opportunity is between the OT practitioner and the community. Community in this relationship includes the populations and settings outside of the client and care team relationships. This also includes professional organizations.

Increasing public understanding of occupational therapy and engaging proactively with key external organizations to assert occupational therapy leadership in areas of societal need is essential to the success of the occupational therapy profession (AOTA, 2013). The relationship with the community and the impact that occupational therapy can have on external stakeholders is key to the future of the profession. As always, membership in occupational therapy professional associations, such as AOTA and state associations, is one way to initiate the relationship with the community, as membership and "strength in numbers" can have a larger impact on community and legislation. In addition, volunteer opportunities in unique community settings related to occupational therapy can raise the power of occupational therapy; examples include participation in community organizations that support populations that are common in occupational therapy practice, including those focusing on children and youth with autism or developmental delay, the bullying of adolescents, chronic illness in the adult population, or aging-in-place with the senior population. An OTA also has many opportunities to volunteer in AOTA and NBCOT activities (Tables 2-1 and 2-2), as well as in state association activities.

An occupational therapy practitioner can also participate in non-occupational therapy organizations to network. Examples include membership in Big Brothers or Big Sisters or in the Association of Junior Leagues International, an organization committed to promoting volunteerism, developing the leadership potential of women, and improving communities through effective action and leadership.

TABLE 2-1
AOTA LEADERSHIP ACTIVITIES FOR OTAs

AOTA SUGGESTED ACTIVITIES	CRITERIA FOR PARTICIPATION
AOTA Board of Directors • President, Secretary, Treasurer • Board Director and six directors, elected by the AOTA membership	• Board of Directors: at least 10 years as an OTA
Representative Assembly (RA) • Speaker, Vice Speaker, Recorder, Agenda Chair, BPPC Chair, Representative, and Alternative Representative • OTA Representative and OTA Alternative Representative to the Assembly • Nominating Committee: at least five and not more than nine voting members • Recognition Committee: four members in addition to Chairperson	• Board: OTAs can be board members • OTA Representative: OTA only • Nominating: one voting member must be an OTA • Recognition: one member must be an OTA
Assembly of Student Delegates Chairperson	• Must be an OTA student
Commission of Education (COE) • Commission Education Chair • COE member	• Chair: at least 5 years of experience as an OTA • Member: must be an OTA educator
Commission of Practice (COP) • COP Chair • COP member	• Chair and member: at least 5 years experience as an OTA • Member: must include at least one OTA
Ethics Commission (EC) • EC Chair • EC OTA member	• Chair: must be initially certified as OTA • Member: must be an OTA
Special Interest Sections (SIC) • Special Interest Section Chair (multiple sections available)	• Chair: at least 5 years experience as an OTA

Note: The AOTA allows OT and OTAs to identify specific volunteer opportunities through a volunteer profile to match the area(s) of expertise, years of experience, amount of time available for volunteering, and other criteria. Not all available opportunities are listed above.

Adapted and abbreviated from AOTA's *Cool! The Volunteer Database* (2014) at http://www.aota.org/AboutAOTA/Get-Involved/Leadership/COOL.aspx.

Table 2-2
NBCOT Leadership Activities for OTAs

NBCOT SUGGESTED ACTIVITIES	CRITERIA FOR PARTICIPATION
• Item Writer Program • Help to develop examination items for the COTA examinations	• Current COTA certification • 3 to 5 years of experience in a specific occupational therapy practice area including mental health, physical disabilities, pediatrics, school-based
• Certification Examination Validation Committee • Serve on a committee that reviews and validates the OTR or COTA examinations	• Good writing, reviewing, and editing skills • Commitment to work within a scheduled timeline • Ability to work well in teams • Computer literate • Willing and able to travel to meetings if necessary

Adapted and abbreviated from NBCOT: http://www.nbcot.org/certificant-volunteering

Note: Volunteering with NBCOT offers an opportunity to give back to the OT profession and an opportunity to network with peers and provide personal and professional recognition. Not all available opportunities are listed above.

Summary

Occupational therapy practitioners are constantly interacting with people and creating relationships where there are numerous chances to become better leaders. Opportunities arise in four primary relationships, including those that an occupational therapy practitioner has with himself or herself, the client, the interdisciplinary care team, and the community. Occupational therapy practitioners have the ability to be creative when generating leadership opportunities within these relationships and can be leaders in the occupational therapy profession without being in an authoritative role.

There are implications that these relationships and future leadership opportunities will evolve as the power of technology continues to emerge in OT education, social media, and health care delivery. Positive effects of technology may lead to the increased accessibility and ease of leadership activity involvement. These include, but are not limited to, optimizing the self-reflection process (relationship with self), service delivery in telehealth (relationship with the client), networking and virtual education (relationship with the interdisciplinary care team), and social media for advocacy of occupational therapy (relationship with the community). Table 2-3 identifies suggested leadership activities within each of these relationships.

ADVOCACY

Advocacy is the process of supporting a cause, such as an idea, policy, or activity, that can directly affect a person's or group's well-being. The role of advocacy in occupational therapy is necessary not only for the strength of the profession, but also for optimum care for clients. This

TABLE 2-3	
ACTIVITIES TO PROMOTE LEADERSHIP IN PRIMARY OCCUPATIONAL THERAPY RELATIONSHIPS	
RELATIONSHIP WITH SELF	**RELATIONSHIP WITH THE CLIENT**
Center of model; the OTA must understand his or her strengths, weaknesses, goals, and motivators	*Occurs in everyday practice; includes relationship with a person, group, or population*
Activities that promote leadership: • Self-reflection each semester or every 6 months • Interview preparation and practice • Professional goal writing • Participation in AOTA Emerging Leaders program	Activities that promote leadership: • Providing unique service delivery or education strategy • Incorporating evidence-based practice; staying current • Connecting families to support group, or starting a support group • Obtaining AOTA Board or Specialty Certifications
RELATIONSHIP WITH THE INTERDISCIPLINARY TEAM	**RELATIONSHIP WITH THE COMMUNITY**
Includes members of the team who are assuming responsibility of a client's care	*Includes the populations and settings outside of the client and care team relationships*
Activities that promote leadership: • Interdisciplinary team rounds • Communication and collaboration through publication (e.g., another discipline's journal) • Communication and collaboration through presentation (e.g., meetings, in-services)	Activities that promote leadership: • Volunteer opportunities in unique community settings related to OT • Participation in non-OT organizations to network, gain stakeholders, and spread OT mission • Advocacy efforts at state and federal levels • Membership in professional organizations

aspect of the chapter defines advocacy and the organizations that support advocacy efforts for occupational therapy practitioners. It also highlights the benefits of occupational therapy advocacy and identifies advocacy activities at the state and federal levels.

Federal and State Advocacy

The AOTA is the national professional organization in the United States that "is responsible for guiding and developing professional standards, professional development and advocacy on behalf of occupational therapy practitioners and the clients serviced by occupational therapy" (Phillips, 2014, p. 1008). Membership in this organization as a student or practitioner should be inherent, as the success of the profession, including professional standards and advocacy, is represented by the number of members. Joining as a student and remaining a lifelong member will demonstrate a commitment to practice and ongoing professional development.

An integral part of the provision of occupational therapy services is the implementation of health policy related to occupational therapy at the federal level. Health policy is a written statement that describes the intended course of an issue related to health. At the state and federal level, political action committees can be used to increase support for health policy legislation. A political action committee provides funding to state and federal candidates who support a profession or industry and their initiatives through private donations from association members. AOTPAC is for AOTA members. Contributions to AOTPAC are optional but can only be accepted by AOTA members. AOTPAC is able to support congressional candidates who support occupational therapy legislation, specifically following the implementation of the Patient Protection and Affordable Care Act in 2010 (see Chapter 1).

Most states have their own professional occupational therapy association. Membership to the state association in which an OT practitioner is licensed, in addition to AOTA membership, will assist with support of the profession at the state level. Some states also have a political action committee, so it is important for the OT practitioner to know, understand, and belong to the appropriate associations related to occupational therapy. State associations are independent from AOTA but work together to advance the profession. For example, AOTA provides position statements, practice guidelines, and language for occupational therapy, but the state association must work to get these positions, guidelines, and verbiage into state legislation/licensure (Phillips, 2014).

Advocacy Activities in Occupational Therapy

There are many ways to be an advocate for occupational therapy outside of financial contributions to AOTPAC and membership in AOTA or state occupational therapy associations. In fact, participation in advocacy events can be exhilarating and energizing not only for the clinician, but also for the profession. Table 2-4 highlights specific advocacy activities, both formal and informal, in which an occupational therapy practitioner or occupational therapy student can participate to highlight the value of occupational therapy within society. The case study highlighted earlier in this chapter incorporates a clinician's positive experience while advocating for the occupational therapy profession.

Attending AOTA's annual Hill Day is one activity that has proven rewarding for many practitioners and students in attendance. The event is held on Capitol Hill in Washington, DC and there is the possibility of participating virtually. The purpose of the event is to join other occupational therapy practitioners and students to advocate for the profession and communicate the distinct value of occupational therapy to federal legislators. The event consists of advocacy training, legislation updates, and personal meetings with legislators. Participation in this event can increase confidence in public speaking, which is an important skill for all OT practitioners and students.

Importance of Advocacy for Occupational Therapy

It is critical that OT practitioners understand the importance of advocacy as a professional skill and being an advocate as an ongoing life role to promote the profession. Collaborating with external stakeholders to develop advocacy skills and participation in advocacy activities can increase awareness and understanding to the importance of advocacy (Hammel, Charlton, Jones, Kramer, & Wilson, 2014). There are some key areas in which both state OT associations and AOTA are active for individual members and the profession. These major areas include, but are not limited to:

- Obtaining a strong relationship with policymakers at the federal and state levels
- Constant advocacy efforts with lobbyists and other rehabilitation services
- Ongoing public awareness through community outreach
- Increased training and funding for professional development, including continuing education, professional conferences, and leadership development programs

TABLE 2-4
FORMAL AND INFORMAL ADVOCACY ACTIVITIES FOR OTAs AND OTA STUDENTS

FORMAL:

- Attending AOTA Hill Day and your state's Hill Day (if it does not exist, network with other OT practitioners to create one)
- Representation as an AOTPAC Region Director or Advisor
- Financial contribution to AOTPAC and state's PAC, if applicable
- Meeting with legislators in your home district office
- Attendance at state OT association meetings
- Becoming a "AOTA COOL Volunteer" (see suggested websites)
- Serving on a committee to help at conference or Hill Day
- Running for Association leadership roles (see Table 2-2)

INFORMAL:

- Writing or calling your Representative for support (template available at aota.org)
- Voting for officers of AOTA and state association
- Informing your state representative regarding your concerns
- Keeping informed of current issues via AOTA emails and subscriptions to AOTA blogs
- Keeping your colleagues updated with ongoing legislative efforts

- Promotion of evidence-based practice through publications such as the *American Journal of Occupational Therapy, OT Practice,* and online AOTA blogs
- Support for licensure renewal and ethical practice guidelines (AOTA, 2009)

CONCLUSION

Leadership is a powerful and necessary component for practice for all occupational therapy practitioners. The importance of understanding common leadership theories, effective leadership skills, and activities in the various environments that foster leadership development will allow an occupational therapy practitioner to become a better leader. In addition, the participation in advocacy events is one strong, important role of an OTA, not only for leadership development, but also for the strength of the profession in legislation.

Occupational therapy practitioners are constantly interacting with people and creating relationships where there are numerous chances to become better leaders. Opportunities arise in four primary relationships, including the those that an occupational therapy practitioner has with himself or herself, with the client, with the interdisciplinary care team, and with the community. Occupational therapy practitioners have the ability to be creative when generating leadership opportunities within these relationships and can be leaders in the occupational therapy profession without being in an authoritative role. Table 2-4 identifies suggested leadership activities within each of these relationships.

Advocacy is the process of supporting an idea, policy, or activity that can directly affect a person's well-being. Advocacy in the occupational therapy profession is necessary not only for the strength of the profession, but also for increasing the services provided and resources available that can benefit clients. AOTA is the national professional organization representing occupational therapy in the United States, directly responsible for developing professional standards on behalf of OT practitioners and the clients served. AOTPAC is the political action committee of AOTA that provides financial support to congressional candidates who support occupational therapy legislation. Lifelong membership in AOTA and state associations is essential for the success of the profession and ongoing professional development.

It is easier than one might think to get involved in occupational therapy advocacy efforts. Networking with OT practitioners who are associated with AOTA, AOTPAC, and state associations can also be an excellent resource for ongoing advocacy efforts. Participation in state and federal OT organizations such as AOTA and AOTPAC is a great way to network and connect occupational therapy to the community.

SUGGESTED WEBSITES

- National Board for Certification in Occupational Therapy Self-Assessment tools: http://www.nbcot.org/self-assessment
- NBCOT Volunteer and Stay Connected: http://www.nbcot.org/certificant-volunteering
- American Occupational Therapy Association OTA Leadership Development Toolkit: http://www.aota.org/otatoolkit
- AOTA Cool! The Volunteer Database: http://www.aota.org/cool
- AOTA Advocacy and Policy (includes AOTPAC): http://www.aota.org/Advocacy-Policy.aspx

REVIEW QUESTIONS

1. Which of the following statements is not true?
   a. Leadership is the practice of encouraging others to purposefully accomplish an outcome that will achieve the fullest potential of the individual, department, profession, or community.
   b. The definition of leadership may vary in different professions.
   c. Only people in managerial roles can be leaders.
   d. All occupational therapy practitioners must be leaders, even if the job title does not entail it.

2. Leaders who use a transformational leadership style would most likely do which of the following?
   a. Create strong connections with colleagues that inspire and motivate to achieve goals
   b. Encourage an open dialogue related to personal goals, strengths, and weaknesses
   c. Establish outcomes that exceed extrinsic motivation
   d. All of the above

3. Which of the following statements is true about emotional intelligence?

   a. Emotional intelligence is a skill you are born with—it cannot be learned.

   b. People with a high IQ also have high emotional intelligence.

   c. Emotional intelligence is the ability to perceive, access, generate, and regulate emotions to promote emotional and intellectual growth.

   d. Emotional intelligence is only important in managerial roles.

4. Erin is an OTA finishing her first year in practice. During self-reflection, Erin decides that she can improve her skills in the area of cognition. Recognizing that this is an area of improvement and her goal is to improve this skill set, she finds a continuing education course to fit her needs. Erin is demonstrating which of the following skills?

   a. Self-awareness

   b. Self-regulation

   c. Motivation

   d. None of the above

5. Erin finds out in a staff meeting that, because of budget constraints, her continuing education course registration fee in 6 months will no longer be covered by the department. She is frustrated, but controls her emotions and decides she will still go and will plan accordingly. Her ability to manage her emotions and channel them in a useful way is an example of what leadership skill?

   a. Self-awareness

   b. Self-regulation

   c. Motivation

   d. None of the above

6. When Erin returns from her course, she decides to provide an in-service to her colleagues regarding what she learned about new evidence-based interventions. She describes her desire to work with her supervising OT to implement this intervention and write a case study on her findings. Her supervising OT is thrilled, and wants to learn more about this intervention strategy, prompting her to pursue her own literature search. What is the main leadership characteristic that Erin is displaying?

   a. Self-awareness

   b. Self-regulation

   c. Motivation

   d. All of the above

7. There are four relationships discussed in this chapter that OT practitioners are a part of that can promote leadership opportunities. Which of the following statements is true?

   a. An OT practitioner must have a good understanding of his or her strengths, weaknesses, goals, and motivators to be a leader.

   b. Self-reflection and knowledge of one's strengths and weaknesses can increase leadership potential.

   c. The process of professional development begins early in the career of an OTA beginning with self-reflection during school.

   d. All of the above

8. The role of an occupational therapy practitioner on the interdisciplinary care team is important for which of the following reasons?

    a. Interdisciplinary teams are more effective than control groups for increasing patient outcomes and satisfaction and decreasing lengths of stay for certain populations.

    b. The relationship between an occupational therapy practitioner and the members of the interdisciplinary team is important for advocacy of the occupational therapy profession.

    c. Some disciplines don't know the role of occupational therapy practitioners.

    d. All of the above

9. Kim is in the final year of her OTA education and wants to become more involved in federal advocacy. Which activities would be appropriate for Kim to participate in to meet her needs?

    a. Writing a letter to her state legislator requesting his or her support on an upcoming bill

    b. Participating in AOTA Hill Day virtually

    c. Becoming a member of her state association and encouraging classmates to do the same

    d. All of the above

10. Which definition best describes the role of a political action committee (PAC)?

    a. A PAC is a group of people who organize fundraisers for a professional organization.

    b. The purpose of a PAC is to draft legislation for state and federal legislators.

    c. A PAC provides funding to state and federal candidates who support a profession and initiatives through private donations from association members.

    d. The purpose of a PAC is to make sure that legislators who do not support occupational therapy are not elected.

REFERENCES

Aarons, G. (2006). Transformational and transactional leadership: Association with attitudes towards evidence-based practice. *Psychiatric Services, 57,* 1162-1169.

American Occupational Therapy Association (2009). *Why be involved? What do my state association and AOTA do for me?* Retrieved from http://www.aota.org/-/media/Corporate/Files/Practice/OTAs/OTA-Leadership/Benefits/20%20-%20Why%20Be%20Involved.pdf

American Occupational Therapy Association. (2013). 2017 and beyond: Mile marker on the road to the Centennial Vision. *AOTA Annual Report 2012–2013.* Bethesda, MD: AOTA Press.

American Occupational Therapy Association. (2014). Occupational therapy practice framework: Domain and process (3rd ed.). *American Journal of Occupational Therapy, 68*(Suppl. 1).

Goleman, D. (1998, November/December). What makes a leader? Best of HBR 1998. *Harvard Business Review,* 4-13. Available at: http://leadershipgovernancemanagementbank.com/wp-content/uploads/2013/03/Tesse-Akpeki-WhatMakesaLeader.pdf

Hammel, J., Charlton, J., Jones, R. Kramer, J., & Wilson, T. (2014). Disability rights and advocacy. In B. Boyt Schell, G. Gillen, & M. Scaffa (Eds.), *Willard & Spackman's occupational therapy* (pp. 1031-1050). Baltimore, MD: Lippincott Williams & Wilkins.

Hand, C., Law, M., & McCool, M. (2011). Occupational therapy intervention for chronic illness: A scoping review. *American Journal of Occupational Therapy, 65,* 428-436.

Mayer, J., & Salovey, P. (1997). What is emotional intelligence? In P. Salovey & D. Sluyter (Eds.), *Emotional development and emotional intelligence: Implication for educators* (pp. 3-31). New York: Basic Books.

Phillips, S. (2014). Occupational therapy professional organization. In B. Boyt Schell, G. Gillen, & M. Scaffa (Eds.), *Willard & Spackman's occupational therapy* (pp. 1005-1013). Baltimore, MD: Lippincott Williams & Wilkins.

Snodgrass, J. (2011). Leadership development. In K. Jacobs & G. McCormack (Eds.), *The occupational therapy manager* (5th ed., pp. 265-279). Bethesda, MD: AOTA Press.

3

Credentialing

Karen Brady, DEd, OTR/L and Lisa Burns, PhD, OTR/L

ACOTE Standard explored in this chapter:

- B.7.3. Demonstrate knowledge of applicable national requirements for credentialing and requirements for licensure, certification, or registration under state laws.

KEY VOCABULARY

Accredited Occupational Therapy Assistant (OTA) program: One that meets standards established by the ACOTE.

Certification: Process of meeting eligibility requirements for and passing the national certification examination.

Credentialing: Process of assessing and confirming the qualifications of a licensed or certified health care practitioner.

License, registration: State or jurisdiction documentation indicating permission to practice.

Standards of Practice: Requirements that OTAs must follow in the delivery of occupational therapy services.

OTAs trained in the United States must meet several specific requirements in order to practice. The requirements include graduating from an OTA program accredited by the Accreditation Council for Occupational Therapy Education (ACOTE). They also include passing the nationally recognized entry-level exam and fulfilling state requirements for licensure, certification, or registration. OTAs must abide by all applicable stipulations, whether they stem from federal or state leg-

Jacobs K, ed.
Management and Administration for the OTA:
Leadership and Application Skills (pp 33-44).
© 2016 Taylor & Francis Group.

CASE STUDY

ABIGAIL'S JOURNEY

There are specific requirements that OTAs must meet to practice in the United States. These include graduating from an accredited school, passing the national exam, and fulfilling all state requirements. This case study presents the fictional experience of 'Abigail' as she becomes a certified occupational therapy assistant (COTA). After reading the case study, you may wish to refer back to the chapter where specific aspects of the case are described.

Abigail Chooses Occupational Therapy as a Career

When Abigail was in high school, her grandmother was hospitalized after having a stroke. During hospital visits, Abigail came to know the OTA who worked with her grandmother. As she watched her grandmother regain lost skills that were important to her (including the ability to eat, bathe, and dress independently), Abigail realized that she, too, wished to have a profound, positive influence on others. She determined that she would pursue a career as an OTA.

Educational Requirements

Abigail soon learned that the first step toward fulfilling her goal was to earn an associate's degree in occupational therapy. She investigated schools in her home state of Colorado, applied, and was accepted into an accredited 2-year program at a community college. Her formal course work included courses in anatomy and physiology, kinesiology, psychology, and occupation analysis. In addition, she was required to successfully complete three fieldwork rotations: one introductory Level I and two full-time Level II experiences. The fieldwork coordinator at the college explained that fieldwork is usually performed in hospitals, nursing homes, rehabilitation centers, and schools under the direct supervision of a licensed or regulated OTA or occupational therapist (OT). While accreditation standards mandate completion of at least 16 weeks of full time Level II fieldwork (generally two 8-week rotations), Abigail's OTA program required completion of two 10-week Level II rotations.

National Requirements: NBCOT Examination

After successfully completing her program's academic and fieldwork requirements, Abigail received her OTA degree; the next step was to pass the NBCOT exam. She was eligible for the exam because she was in compliance with the Code of Conduct, and she had graduated from an accredited OTA program. Abigail chose to attend an exam review course and took some online practice tests. When she felt ready for the 4-hour exam, she scheduled an exam date with a nearby Prometric testing center. She was elated when, a few weeks later, she received notification that she had passed the exam. The final step was to apply for a license to begin practicing as an OTA.

Licensure

Abigail entered her educational program in 2012. At that time, Colorado did not require OTA licenses. After checking www.colorado.gov/dora/licensing for current information, however, Abigail learned that after June 1, 2014, OTAs in Colorado must complete a license application and receive approval before they can practice. Abigail submitted all the required

(continued)

CASE STUDY (CONTINUED)

documents (including her proof of passing the NBCOT examination) and received her license to practice as an OTA in Colorado.

Summary

Abigail achieved her dream of becoming an OTA. The journey required her to earn an associate's degree, pass the national certification exam, and obtain a Colorado license. She is now working in a rehabilitation facility under the supervision of an OT. While she is not required to complete continuing education to renew her Colorado OTA license, she does plan to maintain her NBCOT certification and is thus following the board's rules regarding re-certification and continuing education. Abigail is planning to pursue specialty certification in low vision (SCALV).

islation, local or specific facility requirements and guidelines, or professional standards. The OTA must be fully informed of all requirements governing his or her practice. This chapter addresses credentialing and the process by which the OTA adheres to applicable national requirements for credentialing and requirements for licensure, certification, or registration under state laws.

GRADUATING FROM AN ACCREDITED OCCUPATIONAL THERAPY ASSISTANT PROGRAM

To practice as an OTA, the individual must first earn an associate's degree from an accredited OTA educational program. An accredited OTA program is one that meets standards established by the American Occupational Therapy Association's (AOTA) ACOTE—formerly known as the AOTA Accreditation Committee. For more than five decades, academic OTA programs have been approved or accredited by the ACOTE or its predecessor. There are currently 205 accredited programs offering the OTA degree at locations throughout the United States, with high concentrations of programs in Florida, Texas, Ohio, and Pennsylvania (AOTA, 2014b, 2014f, 2014g). The accreditation process is designed to both ensure the quality of the program and assist with improving quality. Accreditation of the program benefits not only students, but also faculty, employees, and the general public. Curricula within OTA programs may vary, but each program must initially meet and then remain compliant with established ACOTE standards (AOTA, 2012a). Programs are subsequently reevaluated by ACOTE every 5, 7, or 10 years (AOTA, 2014b). While some accredited programs may offer portions of the curriculum in online or distance education format, there are currently no OTA programs offered entirely online (AOTA, 2014a).

MEETING NATIONAL REQUIREMENTS: THE CERTIFICATION EXAMINATION

In the United States, a person who wishes to practice as an OTA must first become certified. The legislation mandating this requirement in Hawaii becomes effective January 2017 (AOTA, 2014f). Achieving certification means that the OTA candidate has met all eligibility requirements for and has passed the exam administered by the National Board for Certification in Occupational

Therapy (NBCOT). Passing the national certification exam certifies the candidate and entitles him or her to use the certified occupational therapy assistant (COTA) credential. The mission of NBCOT (n.d.) is to "serve the public interest by advancing client care and professional practice through evidence-based certification standards and the validation of knowledge essential for effective practice in occupational therapy." The purpose of the exam is to protect the public interest by certifying only those candidates who possess the knowledge necessary for occupational therapy practice.

Construction of the national certification exam is based on results of practice analysis studies that identify the domains, tasks, and knowledge required for occupational therapy practice. The exam, consisting of 200 multiple choice questions, is designed to measure entry-level competence of candidates who have met exam eligibility requirements. Candidates are allotted 4 hours to complete the exam, which is presented in an electronic format delivered at testing centers throughout the United States. The testing centers are administered by a company called Prometric, a well-established test development and delivery provider. Graduates of accredited OTA programs who are eligible to take the NBCOT certification exam and have completed the registration process will receive an Authorization to Test (ATT) letter. Upon receipt of the ATT letter, candidates may contact any Prometric testing center to schedule an appointment to take the exam (for further information, go to www.Prometric.com).

Exam scores range from 300 to 600 points; these raw scores are scaled to represent equivalent levels of achievement regardless of exam version. Successful exam candidates must achieve a minimum of 450 points. The board provides reasonable and appropriate accommodations for all qualified candidates with a disability who submit appropriate documentation (NBCOT, n.d.).

Certification Exam Eligibility

The NBCOT will accept only candidates who have graduated from either an accredited OTA program within the United States or a program outside of the United States approved by the World Federation of Occupational Therapy (WFOT); currently, no such programs exist. Candidates must have completed all requirements for the OTA degree (including fieldwork) and are required to provide the NBCOT with their official final academic transcript that notes the degree conferral date. In lieu of the final transcript, candidates may temporarily provide an Academic Credential Verification Form, but the NBCOT will not release their exam results until the transcript (indicating degree conferral) is received.

All NBCOT exam candidates must answer questions about their character and agree to abide by the NBCOT Code of Conduct (available at www.nbcot.org). It is in the exam candidates' best interest to be familiar with the code's 8 Principles, as failure to follow the principles can disqualify a person from practicing occupational therapy. For example, Principle 5 includes the stipulation that certain criminal convictions can render one ineligible to sit for the certification exam and, thus, unable to practice. An individualized Early Determination and Character Review is available (for a fee) from the NBCOT; this service enables candidates to learn their eligibility status prior to exam registration (NBCOT, n.d.).

In addition to abiding by the Code of Conduct, applicants must agree to abide by the NBCOT Professional Practice Standards (PPS) at all times. The PPS consists of four sections: Practice Domains, Code of Professional Conduct (described previously), Supervision, and Documentation. The board clarifies that the three-fold intention of PPS is to assist clients in understanding what to expect from a COTA certificant and assist the COTA in understanding his or her role in the delivery of client care and services and in understanding the professional expectations of being certified by the NBCOT (NBCOT, 2014b, 2014c).

TABLE 3-1	
NBCOT PROFESSIONAL DEVELOPMENT UNIT ACTIVITIES CHART	
PROFESSIONAL DEVELOPMENT ACTIVITY	**PDU VALUE**
Attending employer-provided, workplace continuing education	1 hr = 1 unit
Attending approved workshops, seminars, lectures, conferences	1 hr = 1 unit
Completing academic courses related to practice area	1 hr = 1 unit
Receiving mentoring from a certified OT practitioner	2 hrs = 1 unit
Partial sampling; see complete list and details at www.nbcot.org	

Preparing to Take the Certification Exam

Resources are available to assist candidates in preparing for the national certification exam. Academic institutions often make exam review sessions available to their students. Additional resources (including review books, study guides, practice exams, and review courses) are also available through the AOTA, NBCOT, and various companies.

Maintaining National Certification

Successful exam candidates are certified for an initial 3-year period. Periodic renewal is necessary for the NBCOT certification to remain in effect, and a renewal application and fee are required. In addition, OTAs must accrue 36 Professional Development Units (PDUs) in the 3-year period between their initial certification and their renewal due date; the PDUs provide evidence of the assistant's ongoing education and development. The NBCOT provides a chart listing acceptable PDU activities, and an online calculator for converting Continuing Education Units to PDUs. In general, one contact hour earned through successfully completed workshops, seminars, online courses, or conferences (which include an assessment component and are offered by approved providers) is equal to 1.25 PDUs. The PDUs may not be accrued from activities that are a regular part of the OTA's current work role (NBCOT, 2014a). Table 3-1 provides a sampling of PDU activities and values. This PDU requirement for NBCOT certification renewal is separate from continuing education requirements that may be imposed by state or jurisdiction occupational therapy associations.

OTAs renewing their certification must also agree to continue to abide by both the NBCOT Code of Conduct and the PPS (NBCOT, 2014b, 2014c). While initial certification is required for practice throughout the United States, maintenance (renewal) of certification is not mandatory in all states and thus might be considered optional in some cases. Employers of OTAs may, however, require maintenance of certification even when it is not state mandated.

MEETING STATE OR JURISDICTION REQUIREMENTS

In addition to graduating from an accredited OTA program and attaining national certification, occupational therapy assistants must meet state or jurisdiction requirements in order to practice. Occupational therapy practice is regulated in various ways by state laws; varying terms are used to refer to individuals who have met the state's requirements and received permission to practice. Depending on the state, one may need a license, permit, authorization, or registration in order to practice.

At the time of this writing, Guam, Puerto Rico, the District of Columbia, and all states except New York have enacted some form of licensure law for occupational therapy assistants. While New York does not require that OTAs be licensed, the state's legislation does regulate their practice and requires that practitioners be initially certified. Regardless of the specific requirement or term used to indicate permission to practice, all jurisdictions and states except Hawaii currently regulate the practice of occupational therapy assistants; Hawaii will begin regulation of OTAs effective January 1, 2017 (AOTA, 2014c). It is against the law to practice as an OTA unless the state requirements are met and permission to practice has been granted (via license, permit, authorization, or registration).

As described earlier, all states mandate (or, in the case of Hawaii, will mandate in 2017) that OTAs be initially certified with the NBCOT. In addition, individuals wishing to obtain permission to practice must complete an application, pay a fee, and provide supporting documents to the state or jurisdiction occupational therapy organization. Supporting documents may include an official academic transcript, a passport-type photograph, letters of reference, an official certification exam score report (available from the NBCOT), and other documents.

Some states grant permission for an OTA to begin practicing prior to taking the certification exam. Terms such as *temporary license* and *limited permit* are used to refer to this special permission. When this permission is granted, it is usually for a limited time and it may be revoked if the individual does not successfully pass the certification exam. Temporary permission to practice also requires an application, fee payment, and other supporting documents (such as the NBCOT Confirmation of Examination, Registration, and Eligibility to Examine Notice).

Securing state permission to practice (whether temporary or permanent) is a distinct process separate from becoming nationally certified through the NBCOT. The AOTA provides online information about each state's specific requirements under its Education and Careers tab (see "Get/Maintain Your License"). Since the two processes may include similar steps (such as submitting an official final academic transcript), individuals wishing to practice as OTAs must take care to satisfy requirements of both entities.

State legislation, as well as professional, the NBCOT, and employer standards, mandate that OTAs receive supervision from an OT. Supervision is intended to protect public health, safety, and welfare. States vary in how the supervisory requirement is defined (e.g., direct or indirect), carried out, and documented (AOTA, 2009). The OTA should understand that each state has unique supervision requirements, guidelines, and standards (Box 3-1). Questions regarding supervision should be discussed with the supervising OT or clinical supervisor. The OTA may need to contact the state occupational therapy board for official clarification of the question and/or situation (NBCOT, 2014c). In many cases, persons seeking a license or permit to practice as an OTA must include evidence of planned supervision (such as the name and license number of the person who will supervise the OTA) with their application or renewal documents.

Since laws regulating OTAs vary from state to state, it is important to know and abide by the laws specifically governing one's own practice. States and jurisdictions vary not only in how they grant permission to practice and how they regulate supervision, but also in the specific tasks OTAs are permitted to perform. For example, legislation varies concerning the administration of physical agent modalities and the documentation (if any) required to record the practitioner's competence with modalities (AOTA, 2012d).

Maintaining State Permission to Practice

Maintaining one's license, registration, or permit is mandatory if a person wishes to continue to practice as an OTA. The duration that a license, permit, or registration remains valid varies by state from periods of 1 to 3 years. Each state has specific requirements that must be met for a license, registration, or permit to be renewed. These requirements may include an application form, fee payment, evidence of appropriate supervision, evidence of continuing competence or

---

Box 3-1

The COTA should understand that each state has supervision requirements, guidelines, and standards that are unique to that state. If questions and/or situations arise regarding supervision, it is incumbent upon the COTA to discuss his or her question and/or situations with the supervising OT or clinical supervisor. The COTA may need to contact the state occupational therapy board for official clarification of the question and/or situation.

http://www.nbcot.org/practice-standards

---

continuing education, evidence of liability or malpractice insurance coverage, and attestation to abide by various conduct standards and/or abstain from criminal, negligent, unethical conduct (AOTA, 2014e). The OTA will again note similarity between the process for securing or maintaining state permission to practice and the process for achieving or renewing NBCOT certification: both involve a continuing education requirement. While a particular course or activity might be used to satisfy both entities, the OTA must keep in mind that the two processes are separate. The requirement, terminology, and credit allotted for the activity may not be the same for both.

MEETING STANDARDS OF PRACTICE

In addition to meeting national and state requirements, there are standards of practice inherent within the occupational therapy profession. Standards of practice are simply requirements that OTAs must follow in the delivery of occupational therapy services. It is expected that every OTA will follow the profession's practice standards; in some states, regulatory entities specifically reference and require adherence to these standards. Students are introduced to practice standards in their academic education; they become familiar with their application during fieldwork preparation. Official documents provided by the AOTA formally state the profession's practice standards. These documents (such as the *Standards of Practice for Occupational Therapy,* the *Guidelines for Supervision, Roles, and Responsibilities During the Delivery of Occupational Therapy Services,* the *Occupational Therapy Code of Ethics and Ethics Standards,* and others) are available in the Reference Manual of the Official Documents of the American Occupational Therapy Association, Inc. (AOTA, 2014d). The OT candidate will note that the documents' content parallels that of the NBCOT PPS described earlier. These documents, and others found in the *American Journal of Occupational Therapy,* clarify the standards of occupational therapy practice. Additional resources for practice include continuing education courses; many states require accrual of continuing education hours to maintain permission to practice (AOTA, 2012b).

Failure to Uphold National, State, or Professional Standards of Practice

The importance of adhering to national, state, and professional requirements for OTAs cannot be understated. Each entity maintains a system for addressing violations of its standards and a process for investigating complaints. As discussed previously, the NBCOT requires COTAs to abide by the NBCOT Certificant Code of Conduct and PPS. The board, through its Qualification and Compliance Review Committee, may enforce sanctions, probation, suspension, or revocation of certification on those who violate the code. Furthermore, the board reports complaints and NBCOT disciplinary action to the public and state regulatory entities. State regulatory boards, which mandate adherence to professional and ethical standards or codes (they often make use of the AOTA Code and standards) also have a system to discipline occupational therapy assistants who violate regulations or fail to comply with standards. Permission to practice as an OTA may be suspended or permanently revoked by the state entity. Additionally, various sanctions and/or monetary fines may be imposed (Doherty, 2014). The AOTA also has a system to address complaints against its members or members who violate its principles (AOTA, 2010). The association's Ethics Commission implements enforcement procedures for the Code of Ethics; disciplinary actions may include "reprimand, censure, probation, suspension, and permanent revocation of membership" (Doherty, 2014, p. 422).

USING THE OCCUPATIONAL THERAPY ASSISTANT CREDENTIAL

On becoming an OTA, the person becomes entitled to make use of a credential. The U.S. Department of Health and Human Services (2006) defines credentialing as "the process of assessing and confirming the qualifications of a licensed or a certified healthcare practitioner." A credential, then, serves to title and publicly identify an individual who has achieved mastery of particular knowledge or of a practice. The formal credential is usually abbreviated. After graduating from an accredited OTA program, the person will be called an occupational therapy assistant or OTA and can legitimately use the OTA credential. Upon passing the NBCOT exam and achieving certification, the OTA is entitled to use the COTA credential and refer to himself or herself as a certified occupational therapy assistant (note that maintenance of certification with the NBCOT is required for continued use of this credential). While all candidates who pass the exam and maintain certification are entitled to use the credential, practice standards in the practitioner's area dictate whether the certification credential should be used in formal, official, or legal documents (e.g., daily contact notes, progress notes).

In addition to the OTA designation and the COTA credential, there are specialty credentials available through the AOTA to qualified OTAs. These credentials designate certification in or mastery of special knowledge or content areas beyond the assistant's entry-level competence. Specialty certification for assistants (SCA) that may be attained include SCADCM (driving and community mobility), SCAEM (environmental modification), SCAFES (feeding, eating, and swallowing), SCALV (low vision), and SCASS (school systems). OTAs who achieve certification in these areas are eligible to use the specialty credential for 5 years, after which a renewal application (demonstrating continued competence) must be completed (AOTA, 2012c).

OBTAINING FURTHER INFORMATION

The purpose of this chapter was to describe credentialing and the processes by which OTAs abide by national and state requirements for licensure, certification, and registration. As described, OTAs must also follow professional practice requirements (such as those pertaining to practice standards, supervision guidelines, and ethical standards). A variety of resources are available to help OTAs stay apprised of changes that influence their practice. These resources include the NBCOT website, as well as the occupational therapy association Website for each state or jurisdiction. The OTA's academic program, particularly the academic fieldwork coordinator, may also provide information about registering and preparing for the national certification exam and about applying for state permission to practice. The AOTA website provides an outstanding collection of information pertaining to these topics. The site furnishes a list of all accredited OTA programs and contact information for each state or jurisdiction's association. In addition, the site permits AOTA members to access the profession's Official Documents, as well as other resources pertaining to practice, supervision, and ethical standards. Those seeking to learn about the national certification exam and related processes will find general information, NBCOT practice tests, and direct links to the NBCOT.

CONCLUSION

There are several requirements that must be met by OTAs who wish to practice in the United States. This chapter has described those requirements, which range from graduating from an ACOTE-accredited OTA program to meeting national requirements for certification and state stipulations regarding licensure or regulation. It is the professional responsibility of the OTA to become familiar with all requirements and then stay abreast of any changes in the profession or legislation that may affect his or her practice.

SUGGESTED WEBSITES

- American Occupational Therapy Association: www.aota.org
- National Board for Certification in Occupational Therapy: www.nbcot.org
- Prometric: www.prometric.com

REVIEW QUESTIONS

1. To practice as an OTA in the United States, candidates must graduate from:
   a. A program approved by the NBCOT
   b. A program accredited by the ACOTE
   c. A program that meets minimal standards established by the American Medical Association (AMA)
   d. A program that is in compliance with the Professional Practice Standards (PPS)

2. Becoming certified for practice as an OTA:
   a. Entails passing the final examination established by the candidate's academic institution
   b. Entails passing the national certification exam administered by the NBCOT
   c. Entitles the candidate to initially use the COTA credential
   d. Both b and c

3. OTA candidates who have been convicted of a crime:
   a. Are always automatically disqualified from becoming OTAs
   b. Must complete a 5-year waiting period before applying to take the national certification examination
   c. Are ineligible to serve on state OTA boards
   d. Should request an Early Determination and Character Review from the NBCOT to find out whether they are eligible to sit for the certification examination

4. Which of the following statements is true regarding the national certification examination?

   a. All candidates must initially pass the exam if they wish to practice in the United States.

   b. Passing the certification exam is optional, depending on the state in which the candidate wishes to practice.

   c. Passing the certification exam is required only if the candidate wishes to practice in Hawaii or New York.

   d. Upon passing the certification exam, candidates achieve lifelong certification status.

5. Which of the following statements is true regarding obtaining state or jurisdiction permission to practice as an OTA?

   a. Once a candidate passes the certification exam, he or she is able to automatically begin practicing.

   b. While all states or jurisdictions regulate the practice of OTAs, they vary somewhat in their use of terms indicating permission to practice and in their specific rules and regulations.

   c. If a candidate provides an official transcript to the NBCOT, he or she may assume that the desired state or jurisdiction has also received the transcript.

   d. No state or jurisdiction will grant a candidate temporary permission to practice prior to that candidate passing the national certification exam.

6. In addition to national and state regulations, there are standards of professional practice that OTAs must follow. These include:

   a. *Standards of Practice for Occupational Therapy*

   b. *Guidelines for Supervision, Roles, and Responsibilities During the Delivery of Occupational Therapy Services*

   c. *Occupational Therapy Code of Ethics and Ethics Standards*

   d. All of the above, as well as the NBCOT's *Professional Practice Standards*

7. Which of the following statements is/are true regarding an OTA who fails to follow standards of practice and national and/or state requirements?

   a. The NBCOT may enforce sanctions, probation, suspension, or revocation of certification against the OTA.

   b. State regulatory boards may discipline the OTA, may suspend or permanently revoke his or her permission to practice, and may impose sanctions and/or monetary fines.

   c. The AOTA may enforce disciplinary actions (including reprimand, censure, probation, suspension, and permanent revocation of membership) against the member OTA.

   d. All of the above are correct.

8. Which credential is the OTA entitled to use (depending on practice standards in his or her area), regardless of whether he or she maintains ongoing certification with the NBCOT?

   a. COTA

   b. COTA/L

   c. OTA

   d. OTR/L

9. Sally finished her final fieldwork and graduated from an ACOTE-accredited OTA program. She is eager to begin practicing as soon as possible. Whom should she contact to find out whether she can obtain a temporary license to begin practicing before she sits for the certification examination?

a. The NBCOT

b. World Federation of Occupational Therapy

c. The state board or association regulating occupational therapy in Sally's state

d. The AOTA

10. Samuel has just moved to Arkansas from Ohio, where he worked for 1 year after graduating from an accredited OTA program and passing the national certification exam. What must he do before he can begin practicing as an OTA in Arkansas?

a. Apply to retake the NBCOT exam

b. Ensure that his AOTA membership and NBCOT certification are up-to-date

c. Provide his official academic transcript to the NBCOT and the state of Arkansas

d. Obtain permission to practice in Arkansas

REFERENCES

American Occupational Therapy Association. (2009). Guidelines for supervision, roles and responsibilities during the delivery of occupational therapy services. *American Journal of Occupational Therapy, 63,* 173-179.

American Occupational Therapy Association. (2010). Occupational therapy code of ethics and ethics standards. *American Journal of Occupational Therapy, 64*(6 Suppl.), S17-S26. http://dx.doi.org/10.5014/ajot.2010.64S17

American Occupational Therapy Association. (2012a). 2011 Accreditation Council for Occupational Therapy Education (ACOTE®) standards. *American Journal of Occupational Therapy, 66,* S6-S74. http://dx.doi.org/10.5014/ajot.2012.66S6

American Occupational Therapy Association. (2012b). 2011 Official documents available from the American Occupational Therapy Association. *American Journal of Occupational Therapy, 66,* 54-55. http://dx.doi.org/10.5014/ajot.2012.66S4

American Occupational Therapy Association. (2012c). *AOTA certification: Board and specialty portfolio process for certification.* Retrieved from http://www.aota.org/Practitioners/ProfDev/Certification.aspx

American Occupational Therapy Association. (2012d). Physical agent modalities. *American Journal of Occupational Therapy, 66,* 578-580. http://dx.doi.org/10.5014/ajot.2012.66S78

American Occupational Therapy Association. (2014a). *Find a school.* Retrieved from http://www.aota.org/Education-Careers/Find-School.aspx

American Occupational Therapy Association. (2014b). *History of AOTA accreditation.* Retrieved from http://www.aota.org/Education-Careers/Accreditation/Overview/History.aspx

American Occupational Therapy Association. (2014c). *Licensure.* Retrieved from http://www.aota.org/en/Advocacy-Policy/State-Policy/StateNews/2014/Hawaii-Enacts-Occupational-Therapy-Licensure-Law-50th-State-to-License-Occupational-Therapists.aspx#sthash.o5CxaI8j.dpuf

American Occupational Therapy Association. (2014d). *The reference manual of the official documents of the American occupational therapy association. Inc., 19th ed.* Bethesda, MD: AOTA Press.

American Occupational Therapy Association. (2014e). *Occupational therapy assistants: Licensure requirements.* Retrieved from http://www.aota.org/-/media/corporate/files/secure/advocacy/licensure/stateregs/qualifications/ota%20qualifications%20and%20licensure%20requirements-july%202014.pdf

American Occupational Therapy Association. (2014f). *OTA programs: Accredited.* Retrieved from http://www.aota.org/en/Education-Careers/Find-School/AccreditEntryLevel/OTAPrograms.aspx

American Occupational Therapy Association. (2014g). *Overview (ACOTE History, Meetings, Members).* Retrieved from http://www.aota.org/Education-Careers/Accreditation/Overview.aspx

Doherty, R. (2014). Ethical practice. In B. Boyt Schell, G. Gillen, & M. Scaffa (Eds.), *Willard & Spackman's occupational therapy* (12th ed., pp. 413-424). Philadelphia: Lippincott Williams & Wilkins.

National Board for Certification of Occupational Therapy. (n.d.). *Mission.* Retrieved from http://www.nbcot.org

National Board for Certification of Occupational Therapy. (2014a). *Certification renewal handbook.* Retrieved from http://www.nbcot.org

National Board for Certification of Occupational Therapy. (2014b). *Code of conduct.* Retrieved from http://www.nbcot.org/certificant-code-of-conduct

National Board for Certification of Occupational Therapy. (2014c). *COTA practice standards.* Retrieved from http://www.nbcot.org/practice-standards

U.S. Department of Health and Human Services. (2006). *Clarification of credentialing and privileging policy.* Retrieved from http://bphc.hrsa.gov/policiesregulations/policies/pin200222.html

4

Reimbursement

Barbara Larson, MA, OTR/L, FAOTA

ACOTE Standard explored in this chapter:
- B.7.4. Demonstrate knowledge of various reimbursement systems (e.g., federal, state, third party, private payer) and documentation requirements that affect the practice of occupational therapy.

KEY VOCABULARY

Prospective Payment System: A method of reimbursement in which Medicare payment is made on a predetermined fixed amount.

Medicaid: A joint federal and state program that helps with medical costs.

Current Procedural Code (CPT): Alphanumeric code used to report health care services and procedures to payers for reimbursement.

Medicare G-codes: Task-based non-billable codes providers must use on all Medicare Part B claims as of July 1, 2013.

Affordable Care Act (ACA) of 2010 (P.L. 111-148): Passage of the act will significantly restructure health care in the U.S. The act mandates increased quality, access, and affordability in health care.

Jacobs K, ed.
Management and Administration for the OTA:
Leadership and Application Skills (pp 45-55).
© 2016 Taylor & Francis Group.

CASE STUDY

The occupational therapy assistant (OTA) works in a skilled nursing facility (SNF) and has been assigned a new client by the occupational therapist (OT). The client is a 74-year-old female, Mrs. Jones, who was hospitalized for a left leg injury. She required surgery and was in the hospital for 6 days for wound healing and infection control. Following discharge from the hospital, Mrs. Jones was admitted to an SNF for rehabilitation. She lives alone and was independent in her activities of daily living (ADLs) and instrumental ADLs (IADLs) prior to injuring her leg. She has a car, which she drives regularly to run errands, attend church, and visit family and friends who live locally. She plans to continue to do so after discharge.

The OT received a physician's order to evaluate Mrs. Jones following her admission to the SNF. The evaluation found that upper extremity strength and range of motion were normal for her age and gender. She did show weakness in her left lower extremity. No cognitive deficits were identified. The OTA participated in the evaluation by assessing Mrs. Jones's ADLs. During the evaluation, the OTA observed Mrs. Jones favoring her left lower extremity, which she reported to the OT. With the information from the OTA, the OT completed the evaluation report.

The OT evaluation results indicated Mrs. Jones was independent in upper extremity dressing and personal hygiene but needed assistance with lower extremity dressing and activities requiring bending to retrieve items off the floor due to weakness in her left leg. Mrs. Jones was also concerned about being able to lift dishes out of her kitchen cupboards and carry items from her microwave to the table. She noted that her son and daughter-in-law wanted to help with grocery shopping and other errands until she was recovered. Mrs. Jones agreed that was a good decision.

The OT and OTA worked together to establish a plan of care.

Health care reimbursement is complex. With the passage of the ACA of 2010 (P.L. 111-148), how payers reimburse for occupational therapy services is being restructured (Fisher & Friesema, 2013). It is critical that occupational therapy practitioners be knowledgeable about both public and private health insurance programs and respective payment systems (AOTA, 2012). Knowledge, thoughtful inquiry, and focusing on the nuances of reimbursement for occupational therapy services will strengthen the practitioner's ability to receive payment for services while providing efficient, affordable client care.

This chapter will address various reimbursement systems and the importance of documentation in securing payment for occupational therapy services. In doing so, occupational therapy practice settings will be identified and different payment systems explored. The implications of the ACA for OTAs will be addressed. The chapter will conclude with a discussion of the importance of ethics in documentation and the need for advocacy in continuing to ensure that occupational therapy services remain a covered entity in health care reimbursement.

PRACTICE SETTINGS

Occupational therapy practitioners work in numerous settings and practice areas. Practice settings include hospitals, outpatient clinics, skilled nursing facilities, home and community settings, schools, industry, and private practice (Holmes & Clark, 2014). Both the OT and the OTA provide services in each setting. Government regulations, policies and procedures, accreditation standards, and billing and payment practices may differ within each setting. Occupational therapy practice areas include pediatrics, school systems, occupational therapy professional education or research, administration and management, work and industry, mental health, developmental disabilities, rehabilitation, geriatrics, orthopedics, acute care, skilled nursing facilities, and home health (National Board for Certification in Occupational Therapy [NBCOT], 2012). Based on data from the NBCOT, the primary practice area of the OTA is in skilled nursing facilities, followed by geriatrics and rehabilitation (NBCOT, 2012). In each setting, occupational therapy practitioners work to enhance the health and wellness of all clients served. Occupational therapy services are provided for the habilitation and rehabilitation of individuals whose disease or disability limits occupational performance (AOTA, 2014). The OT is responsible for all aspects of occupational therapy service delivery. The OTA is an integral part of service delivery and works under the supervision of and in collaboration with the OT (AOTA, 2014). Think about the case study and the role the OTA had in the evaluation of Mrs. Jones. The OTA observed Mrs. Jones guarding her left lower extremity during the ADL evaluation and reported it to the OT. This a client safety issue. Strategies to address this with the client were included in the plan of care. The level of supervision of the OTA is a combination of factors including institutional policies, state licensure laws and regulations, and the requirements of individual payers of occupational therapy services.

HEALTH CARE PAYMENT SYSTEMS

With the complexities in health care reimbursement, it is important for occupational therapy practitioners to be familiar with public and private health insurers, as well as current payment systems (AOTA, 2012). Payment sources include federal and state insurance programs and health plans offered by private insurance companies. Federal health insurance includes Medicare, Social Security Disability, and programs for federal employees, veterans, and railroad workers (Holmes & Clark, 2014). State programs include Medicaid, Children's Health Insurance Plan (CHIP), and Workers' Compensation (Centers for Medicare & Medicaid Services [CMS] n.d.a, n.d.b).

Medicare, the federal health insurance program, pays a portion of health care costs for people aged 65 years and older and for certain people younger than 65 years of age with long-term disabilities (CMS, n.d.c). Medicare was established in 1965 and has four parts: Part A covers hospital inpatient care, Part B covers outpatient care, Part C covers Medicare Advantage, and Part D covers prescription drugs. Occupational therapy is reimbursed under Part B when the service is reasonable and necessary and delivered by a qualified provider (AOTA, 2013a). The client in our case study met the criteria for Medicare coverage. OT services were reimbursed because, first, the services were reasonable and necessary due to the deficits in Mrs. Jones's occupational performance. Second, the OT is a qualified provider under Medicare and the OTA worked under the supervision of the OT.

Medicare uses a Prospective Payment System, a method of reimbursement in which Medicare payment is made on a predetermined fixed amount (Huckfeldt, Sood, Romely, Malchidodi, & Escarce, 2013). Reimbursement for Medicare payment is based on the services of a skilled provider (CMS, 2009c). Under Medicare, the OT is a skilled provider, whereas the OTA is not. The OT must have a provider number to qualify to bill Medicare (CMS, 2009b). The OTA works under the supervision of the OT (CMS, 2009a, 2013). Occupational therapy provides services incident to a referral by a physician or a non-physician practitioner (CMS, 2012).

Medicaid is a joint federal and state program that helps with medical costs for some people with limited income and resources (CMS, n.d.c). Families with dependent children and the elderly, blind, and disabled who are in financial need are eligible for Medicaid. Medicaid programs vary from state to state, but most health care costs are covered if the individual qualifies for both Medicare and Medicaid. Medicaid may be known by different names in different states. The federal government pays states for a specified percentage of expenditures (CMS, n.d.c; U.S. Census Bureau, 2012).

CHIP is a program administered at the state level, providing health care to low-income children whose parents do not qualify for Medicaid. CHIP may be known by different names in different states. The CHIP program may also be known by its former name, the State Children's Health Insurance Program (SCHIP; CMS, n.d.a; U.S. Census Bureau, 2012).

Military health care includes TRICARE and the Civilian Health and Medical Program of the Department of Veterans Affairs, as well as care provided by the Department of Veterans Affairs (U.S. Census Bureau, 2012).

Workers' Compensation is a state-mandated insurance program that provides compensation to employees who suffer job-related injuries and illnesses. Workers' Compensation provides wage replacement and medical benefits to employees injured during employment in exchange for giving up the right to sue the employer for negligence. While the federal government administers a workers' comp program for federal and certain other types of employees, each state has its own laws and programs for workers' compensation (Legal Information Institute, n.d.).

Private insurance is coverage by a health plan provided through an employer or union or purchased by an individual from a private health insurance company. Private health care plans consist of contracts that specify the rules or conditions under which services will be covered. Examples of private health insurance companies are United, Blue Cross Blue Shield, and Preferred One. Occupational therapy services may not be covered consistently in private health care plans (AOTA, n.d.a, n.d.b).

Consideration of network enrollment, coding, billing, and appeals are important aspects of both ensuring inclusion in health plans and securing reimbursement for occupational therapy services (Hinojosa, 2012). Health care is a dynamic entity, and the only constant is change. For occupational therapy to continue to be a covered entity, it is important for practitioners to persist in educating and informing payers on the value of occupational therapy services to health plan beneficiaries. The lobbying efforts of the AOTA and individual state associations have been critical for inclusion and expansion of occupational services in both public and private insurance plans. Think about our case study. The fact that OT continues to be a covered service under Medicare is a direct result of the ongoing lobbying efforts of our professional associations and the practitioners working with them on our behalf.

REIMBURSEMENT

Health care providers are reimbursed through both public and private health insurance plans. Occupational therapy is one of the covered services in these plans, although the level of coverage may differ depending on the plan. Reimbursement consists of the amount or fee paid for a given service rendered. There are different types of fees, including fee-for-service, fee schedules, per diem rates, and a per episode of care rate (Holmes & Clark, 2014).

Fees are based on a formula and may be paid in many different ways. These formulas consist of a relative value unit (RVU) and a monetary conversion factor. Components of the RVU are the following. The conversion factors are determined by geographic cost differences. "Set by agreement between the contractor/facility (provider) of service and the payer, the reimbursement payment is typically determined in advance" (Holmes & Clark, 2014, p. 520).

As stated in the section on health care payment systems, changes in these systems happen frequently, and it is the responsibility of the occupational therapy practitioner to stay informed of these changes.

The Center for Medicare and Medicaid Services Office of Financial Management has identified what a therapist needs to do under Medicare to be reimbursed (CMS, 2012). An individualized plan of care must be written based on the following: evaluation results, establishment of a rehabilitation diagnosis, and specific interventions to be used to address the client's needs. Goals, expected outcomes, and any predicted level of improvement are also included. The intensity, frequency, and duration of care and the anticipated discharge plans are indicated (CMS, 2012). In our case study, Mrs. Jones had an individualized plan of care, which included evaluation results, and a rehabilitation diagnosis related to her occupational performance deficits. The OT and OTA collaborated with the client on setting goals. Both contributed to the intervention plan. Mrs. Jones would have assistance at home. She demonstrated an awareness of her abilities and limitations. It was anticipated that Mrs. Jones would return home following 2 weeks of daily OT sessions.

Medicare continues to be the largest funding agency for reimbursement of occupational therapy services (AOTA, n.d.d). To be reimbursed, the level of complexity of the treatment or the condition of the client requires a skilled service. The service must be performed by a qualified therapist, or in the case of occupational therapy, an OTA under the supervision of a qualified OT (Ramsdell, 2009). The Medicare regulation that defines a qualified OT is §§230.2 (Ramsdell, 2009). Both OTs and OTAs meet Medicare personnel qualifications. OTs can enroll in Medicare as providers of OT services, but OTAs cannot. The services of the OTA are billed through the enrolled therapist or another therapy provider (CMS, 2009c). OTAs under the supervision of the OT may provide skilled and medically necessary services appropriate to each client's plan of care (CMS, 2009a). In the case of Mrs. Jones, the OTA provided a skilled service working on the ADL areas identified in the evaluation. While the OTA could not bill Medicare directly, the OT services could be billed through the OT. This is possible because, when working under the supervision of the OT, the OTA met Medicare personnel qualifications.

It is important to understand Medicare reimbursement, as other payers often follow Medicare in determining guidelines for reimbursement of therapy services. Private payers, while regulated state by state, are required to use U.S. Department of Health and Human Services standards for reimbursement (American Association of Professional Coders, n.d.a). The ACA, addressed in a later section, will impact the Medicare reimbursement of therapy services and subsequently other payers who choose to adopt Medicare guidelines (Fisher & Friesema, 2013).

CODING AND BILLING

Reimbursement is based on claims and documentation filed by providers using medical diagnosis and procedure codes (American Association of Professional Coders, n.d.a). Billing for occupational therapy services requires knowledge of coding. There are three types of codes a practitioner should be familiar with: the International Classification of Diseases, Ninth Revision, Clinical Modification (ICD-9-CM); CPT; and Healthcare Common Procedure Coding System (HCPCS); Centers for Disease Control [CDC], n.d.; Holmes & Clark, 2014).

The ICD-9-CM is the official system of assigning codes to diagnoses and procedures associated with hospital utilization in the United States (CDC, n.d). The physician has the responsibility to determine the diagnosis and assign an ICD-9-CM code. The occupational therapy practitioner determines which procedural codes to use based on the payer and intervention provided to the client. The codes used by the therapist must match the diagnosis assigned by the physician (Holmes & Clark, 2014). The code set is updated at least annually based on the input of providers, payers, and others. A much larger code set, ICD-10-CM, will replace ICD-9 codes on October 1, 2015 (American Association of Professional Coders, n.d.b). In our case study, the physician would determine the diagnosis code (ICD-9-CM) related to the injury Mrs. Jones had to her left leg. The OT would bill Medicare using the appropriate CPT code. The CPT code must relate to the diagnosis code selected by the physician. In Mrs. Jones's case, the OT services billed must address the deficits caused by her leg injury. A code for "self care and home management training" would be appropriate because the deficits she has in ADLs relate directly to her leg injury. If the OT practitioner used the code for the "development of cognitive skills," the claim would be denied.

CPT codes are a listing of standardized descriptions, in numerical form, used to report health care services and procedures to payers for reimbursement. The purpose of CPT is to provide a uniform language accurately describing medical, surgical, and diagnostic services. CPT codes provide an effective means for reliable nationwide communication within the health care industry (American Association of Professional Coders, n.d.b). The American Medical Association owns and copyrights the CPT codes (American Association of Professional Coders, n.d.b). CPT codes are the primary set of codes used by practitioners (CMS, 2009c).

Medicare is now mandating functional limitation reporting and the use of task based G-codes. Moving from an impairment only base—that is, how much improvement there has been in the physical impairment—the Center for Medicare and Medicaid Services has changed its thinking (Doucet, 2014). In mandating a change to task-based G-codes and modifiers on all claims submitted for outpatient Medicare Part B recipients, CMS now reasons that "therapy services should be driven by a person's ability to return to purposeful activities, and not just based on improvement of physical impairment" (Doucet, 2014, p. 123). Think about our case study. Mrs. Jones, due to her leg injury, had difficulty with occupational performance in specific ADL areas. The OT's intervention plan focused on increasing occupational performance in those areas—not on the physical impairment affecting Mrs. Jones.

As of July 1, 2013, to be reimbursed, OTs billing for outpatient therapy services under Medicare Part B are required to use functional reporting on their claims, in the form of non-payable G-codes and modifiers (CMS, 2009a). G-codes identify primary issues being addressed by therapy, and modifiers reflect clients' functional limitations. CMS plans to use the data to track functional change over time (AOTA, 2013a). Looking at functional change in a client related to how this change affects occupational performance is critical to the practice of occupational therapy. Occupational therapy practitioners need to have an understanding of how to use coding correctly. An OTA may be entering G-codes, CPT codes, or HCPCS codes. Incorrect coding may result in denial of payment. In large organizations, there is often a billing office, where individuals are specially trained to handle coding and billing procedures and understand the requirements of different payers. In smaller facilities and many private practices, it is up to the practitioner to make sure that correct codes are used and that all billing is accurate and timely. In addition, keep in mind that other payers often follow Medicare guidelines for payment of therapy services.

DOCUMENTATION

Accurate, timely, focused clinical documentation is a critical component of occupational therapy practice. "Well-documented occupational therapy services are more likely to be recognized and reimbursed as a cost effective treatment in improving health and quality of life" (Gateley & Borcherding, 2012, p. 1). Documentation is part of the medical record and serves as a communication tool among health care providers involved in a client's care. A practitioner's documentation is a legal record and protects the rights of both the client and the therapist. Because it is a legal record, documentation can be used in judicial proceedings such as disability hearings, Workers' Compensation settlements, and court cases. Third-party payers determine whether to pay or deny a claim based on the a documentation submitted by the provider.

Documentation requirements vary among payers, employers, and payment systems. With cost containment a priority in health care, payers are increasing both the scrutiny and the expectations for provider documentation (Jacobs, 2011). It is important that OT practitioners follow the specific guidelines and policies at their current employment setting related to documentation of occupational therapy services (AOTA, 2013b). Written documentation guidelines and policies also apply to electronic health records. With advances in technology, the health care industry is moving toward electronic data management. There are many thoughts on how electronic documentation will contribute to making health care more accessible and affordable. Porter, Lee, and

Thomas (2013) suggest that if an electronic medical record is done correctly, clients will provide one set of information, with a centralized way to schedule appointments and communicate with health care providers. The principles that guide contemporary practice—client centered, occupation centered, and evidence based—should be evident in our documentation (Gateley & Borcherding, 2012).

Documentation should reflect a skilled service has been provided, that is within the occupational therapy scope of practice (AOTA, 2010a). When analyzing client performance in the documentation process, clinical reasoning should be part of the occupational therapy practitioner's reasoning (AOTA, 2013b; Gray, 2014; Lyons & Crepeau, 2001). Researchers have identified several types of clinical reasoning, including procedural, interactive, conditional, narrative, and pragmatic (Lyons & Crepeau, 2001). For example, consider the components of conditional reasoning as it could apply to documenting client performance. As stated by Lyons and Crepeau (2001), "Conditional reasoning is a high-level skill because it synthesizes what the therapist knows about the person, the disease, and the various therapeutic activities that could be employed" (p. 579). Synthesis of information gained and observations made during a treatment session are important considerations during the assessment part of documentation. Clear, focused documentation that demonstrates the necessity of skilled occupational therapy services will meet established criteria for reimbursement of health care insurance plans (CMS, 2009a).

AFFORDABLE CARE ACT

The passage of the ACA, the largest government funding of health insurance since 1965 when Medicare and Medicaid were established, is significantly changing health care in the United States (Fisher & Friesema, 2013; Hinojosa, 2012). Medicare, the largest government-funded health insurance program, is slated for major revisions that will affect beneficiaries. The Medicaid program will also see changes. As other payers commonly follow Medicare, changes will be seen industry wide (Fisher & Friesema, 2013). Payment to health care providers will be restructured (Huckfeldt et al., 2013). Health care providers will be expected to increase their productivity and hold down costs without investing in more resources (Fisher & Freisema, 2013). There will be greater emphasis on efficiency and quality of services.

The AOTA has identified the implications of the ACA for OTAs (AOTA, n.d.c). The OTA has the potential to see an expanding client base due to several factors: the uninsured gaining access to health care, expansion of Medicaid services in some states, new care delivery models, and emphasis on an integrated, team-based approach to providing care (AOTA, n.d.c).

OTAs are encouraged to become advocates for the profession and promote the fact that they are integral to the practice of occupational therapy, provide a skilled service, and are a recognized entity by payers of occupational therapy services (AOTA, n.d.c). Under the ACA, the OTA may see expanded roles. With the expectation for increased productivity with limited resources, there will be a need for partnering with the OT in managing costs and efficiencies (Fisher & Freisema, 2013). OTAs are well positioned to participate in managing and providing information and documentation related to outcome achievement, contributing to policy development, and assisting the OT in implementing strategies for the changes forthcoming in health care in the United States. The OTA also must be a strong advocate for the profession, educating both public and private payers of health care services on the value of occupational therapy to beneficiaries (AOTA, 2009).

ETHICS

Occupational therapy practitioners have an ethical responsibility to those they serve. The AOTA (2010b) has identified seven core ethical concepts for the occupational therapy profession: altruism, equality, freedom, justice, dignity, truth, and prudence. The NBCOT (n.d.), in its *Code of Conduct*, has developed principles that address professional communication with clients, professional colleagues, external audiences, and within the social media environment (NBCOT, n.d.). Ethical decision making requires an awareness of the impact that occupational therapy will have on every client and in every work environment. An example of a possible ethical issue is billing for OT services based on productivity requirements rather than the needs of the clients. The question may become one of deciding the ethics of continuing to see a client and billing for services even if the client no longer requires skilled occupational therapy services. In looking at our case study, once Mrs. Jones has met her OT goals, she no longer requires skilled occupational therapy services. Therefore, she is no longer eligible for OT coverage under Medicare and will be discharged from occupational therapy. Whether an OT or an OTA, we share the same responsibility for ethical practice.

CONCLUSION

Reimbursement is complicated, and it is critical to have an understanding of the payment systems that affect practice. The passage of the ACA is restructuring health care. There is a mandate for increased health care access, affordability, and quality. Productivity expectations are increasing, but resources are not. Practitioners need to understand and plan for these changes. Decisions should be made using facts and based on supporting evidence. Practitioners need to stay committed to the core concepts of occupation-based practice and the evidence that guides our decision making (AOTA, 2010a, 2014). The OTA is well positioned to have an impact on improving the efficiency and affordability of occupational therapy service delivery (AOTA, 2007).

Occupational therapy practitioners can be successful advocates for the profession. The challenge is to stay informed. The AOTA and state occupational therapy associations are excellent resources. One of the critical services they provide is extensive lobbying for inclusion of occupational therapy in both public and private health insurance plans. Attend meetings, and ask questions. Knowledge, advocacy, and action are vital to the continued recognition of occupational therapy as an integral participant in today's ever-changing health care arena.

SUGGESTED WEBSITES

- Centers for Medicare & Medicaid Services: www.cms.gov
- World Health Organization's International Classification of Diseases: www.who.int/classifications/icd/en/
- Centers for Disease Control: www.cdc.gov
- Affordable Care Act: www.hhs.gov/healthcare/rights/law/index.html
- American Occupational Therapy Association, Coverage and Reimbursement: http://www.aota.org/Advocacy-Policy/Federal-Reg-Affairs/Pay.aspx

REVIEW QUESTIONS

1. Identify the primary practice setting where most OTAs work:
    a. Rehabilitation centers
    b. School systems
    c. Skilled nursing facilities
    d. Hospitals

2. The largest payer of health care services in the United States is:
    a. Blue Cross Blue Shield
    b. Medicaid
    c. Medicare
    d. ACA

3. The ICD-9-CM codes are:
    a. Therapy codes
    b. Diagnostic codes
    c. Procedural codes
    d. Incident codes

4. Federal health care insurance plans include:
    a. Medicare, Social Security Disability, Veterans Affairs programs
    b. Workers' Compensation, Medicaid, Social Security Disability
    c. Workers' Compensation, Veterans Affairs programs, CHIP
    d. VA programs, Medicaid, Social Security Disability

5. An RVU includes all of the following except:
    a. Time used by the provider
    b. Quality measurement factors
    c. Expenses of running a practice
    d. Professional liability expenses

6. Which statement best describes private health insurance?
    a. The cost is subsidized by the federal government.
    b. OT coverage is the same as in Medicare.
    c. Examples include Medicaid and Blue Cross Blue Shield.
    d. It can be provided through an employer.

7. The following are codes used by occupational therapy practitioners. Select the codes that are non-billable.
    a. CPT codes
    b. HCPCS codes
    c. G-codes
    d. ICD-9-CM codes

8. The following statement does not accurately describe occupational therapy documentation:

   a. It is a medical record.

   b. It requires a physician's signature.

   c. It can be used in a court of law.

   d. It protects the rights of the OT and client.

9. Which of the following is not reflective of the ACA?

   a. Focuses on access to health care and affordability

   b. Restructures payment to health care providers

   c. Increases and expands provider resources

   d. Emphasizes quality and efficiency of services

10. Under the ACA, the OTA has the potential to:

   a. See an increased client base

   b. Require greater supervision

   c. Supervise OT students

   d. Bill independently

REFERENCES

American Association of Professional Coders. (n.d.a). *What is medical reimbursement?* Retrieved from https://www.aapc.com/resources/medical-coding/reimbursement.aspx

American Association of Professional Coders. (n.d.b). *What is CPT?* Retrieved from https://www.aapc.com/resources/medical-coding/cpt.aspx

American Occupational Therapy Association. (2007). AOTA's Centennial vision and executive summary. *American Journal of Occupational Therapy, 61,* 613-614.

American Occupational Therapy Association. (n.d.a). *Private pay.* Retrieved from www.aota.org/Advocacy-Policy/Federal-Reg-Affairs/Pay/Private.aspx

American Occupational Therapy Association. (n.d.b). *Coding and billing.* Retrieved from http://www.aota.org/en/Advocacy-Policy/Federal-Reg-Affairs/Coding/FAQ.aspx

American Occupational Therapy Association. (n.d.c). *Health care reform and the occupational therapy assistant.* Retrieved from http://www.aota.org/-/media/Corporate/Files/Advocacy/Health-Care-Reform/Overview/HCR_OTA.pdf

American Occupational Therapy Association. (n.d.d). *Coverage and reimbursement.* Retrieved from ttps://www.aota.org/en/Advocacy-Policy/Federal-Reg-Affairs/Pay.aspx

American Occupational Therapy Association. (2009). Guidelines for supervision, roles, and responsibilities during the delivery of occupational therapy services. *American Journal of Occupational Therapy, 63,* 797-803.

American Occupational Therapy Association. (2010a). Scope of practice. *American Journal of Occupational Therapy, 64,* S70-S77. doi:10.5014/ajot.2010.64S70.

American Occupational Therapy Association. (2010b). Occupational therapy code of ethics and ethics standards. *American Journal of Occupational Therapy, 64*(6 Suppl.), S17-S26. doi: 10.5014/ajot.2010.64S17-64S26.

American Occupational Therapy Association. (2012). 2011 Accreditation standards for occupational therapy education (ACOTE) standards. *American Journal of Occupational Therapy, 66*(6 Suppl.), S6-S74. doi:10.5014/ajot.2012.66S6.

American Occupational Therapy Association. (2013a). *Medicare Part B, functional data reporting for CY 2013.* Retrieved from www.aota.org/Advocacy-Policy/Federal-Reg-Affairs/Coding/G-Code.aspx

American Occupational Therapy Association. (2013b). Guidelines for documentation of occupational therapy. *American Journal of Occupational Therapy, 67*(6 Suppl.) S33-S38.

American Occupational Therapy Association. (2014). Occupational therapy practice framework: Domain and process (3rd ed). *American Journal of Occupational Therapy, 68,* S1-S51.

Centers for Disease Control (n.d.). *International classification of diseases, ninth revision, clinical modifications (ICD-9-CM).* Retrieved from http://www.cdc.gov/nchs/icd/icd9cm.htm

Centers for Medicare & Medicaid Services. (2009a). *Covered medical and other health services section 220—coverage of outpatient rehabilitation therapy services (physical therapy, occupational therapy, and speech-language pathology services) under medical insurance.* Retrieved from http://cms.hhs.gov/Regulations-and-Guidance/Guidance/Manuals/downloads/bp102c15.pdf

Centers for Medicare & Medicaid Services.. (2009b). *Covered medical and other health services section 230.2—practice of physical therapy, occupational therapy, and speech-language pathology in Medicare benefit policy manual.* Retrieved from http://cms.hhs.gov/Regulations-and-Guidance/Guidance/Manuals/downloads/bp102c15.pdf

Centers for Medicare & Medicaid Services. (2009c). *11 Part B billing scenarios for OT and PT.* Retrieved from http://www.cms.gov/site-search/search-results.html?q=11%20part%20b%20billing%20scenarios%20for%20pts%20and%20ots

Centers for Medicare & Medicaid Services. (2012). *Preparing for therapy required functional reporting implementation in CY.* National Provider Call, P. R. West. Retrieved from http://www.cms.gov/site-search/search-results.html?q=national%20provider%20cal

Centers for Medicare & Medicaid Services. (n.d.a). *Children's Health Insurance Program (CHIP).* Retrieved from http://www.medicaid.gov/Medicaid-CHIP-Program-Information/By-Topics/Childrens-Health-Insurance-Program-CHIP/Childrens-Health-Insurance-Program-CHIP.html

Centers for Medicare & Medicaid Services. (n.d.b). *Prospective payment system—general information.* Retrieved from http://www.cms.gov/Medicare/Medicare-Fee-for-Service-Payment/ProspMedicareFeeSvcPmtGen/index.html?redirect=/prospmedicarefeesvcpmtgen/04_psf_sas.asp

Centers for Medicare & Medicaid Services. (n.d.c). *Financing and reimbursement.* Retrieved from http://www.medicaid.gov/search.html?q=financing%20and%20reimbursement

Doucet, B. M. (2014). From the desk of the associate editor, quantifying function: Status critical. *American Journal of Occupational Therapy, 68,* 123-126. http://dx.doi.org/10.5014/ajot2014.010991

Fisher, G., & Friesema, J. (2013). Health policy perspectives—implications for the Affordable Care Act for occupational therapy practitioners providing services to Medicare recipients. *American Journal of Occupational Therapy, 67,* 502-506.

Gateley, C. A., & Borcherding, S. (2012). Documentation manual for occupational therapy writing soap notes (3rd ed.). Thorofare, NJ: SLACK Incorporated.

Gray, K. (2014, March). How did billable come to equal productivity, and what do we do now? *Administration & Management Special Interest Section Quarterly, 30*(1), 1–4.

Holmes, D. E., & Clark, L. L. (2014), Laws, credentials and reimbursement. In K. Jacobs, N. MacRae, & K. Slaydk (Eds.), *Occupational therapy essentials for clinical competence* (2nd ed.). Thorofare, NJ: Slack Incorporated.

Hinojosa, J., (2012). The issue is personal strategic plan development. Getting ready for change in our professional and personal lives. *American Journal of Occupational Therapy, 66,* a34-e38. http://dx.doi.org/10.5014/ajot.2012.002360

Huckfeldt, P. J., Sood, N., Romely, J. A., Malchidodi, A., & Escarce, J. J. (2013). Medicare payments reform and provider entry and exit in the post-acute care market. *Health Science Research, 48,* 5. doi:10.111/1475-6773.12059.

Jacobs, K. (2011). Evolution of occupational therapy delivery systems. In K. Jacobs & G. L. McCormack (Eds.), *The occupational therapy manager* (5th ed., pp. 37-50). Bethesda, MD: AOTA Press.

Legal Information Institute. (n.d.). *Workers compensation.* Cornell University Law School. Retrieved from www.law.cornell.edu/wex/workers_compensation

Lyons, K. D., & Crepeau, E. B. (2001). Case report. The clinical reasoning of an occupational therapy assistant. *American Journal of Occupational Therapy, 55*(5), 577-581.

National Board for Certification in Occupational Therapy. (n.d.). *Code of conduct.* Retrieved from http://www.nbcot.org/code-of-conduct

National Board for Certification in Occupational Therapy. (2012). *2012 Practice analysis of the certified occupational therapy assistant.* Retrieved from www.nbcot.org/exam-blueprints

Porter, M. E., Lee, M. E., & Thomas, H. (2013). The strategy that will fix health care. *Harvard Business Review, 91*(10). Retrieved from http://hbr.org/product/the-strategy-that-will-fix-health-care/an/R1310B-PDF-ENG

Ramsdell, R. L. (2009). *Last piece of the puzzle series, Multidisciplinary Academy of Affiliated Medical Arts (MAAMA).* Retrieved from http://www.maama.org/WHO%20CAN%20PROVIDE%20THERAPY%20FOR%20MY%20MEDICARE%20PATIENT.pdf

U.S. Census Bureau. (2012). *Health insurance, CPS health insurance definitions.* Retrieved from https://www.census.gov/hhes/www/hlthins/methodology/definitions/cps.html

5

Marketing and Promoting

Karen Jacobs, EdD, OTR/L, CPE, FAOTA

ACOTE Standards explored in this chapter:

- B.7.5. Demonstrate the ability to participate in the development, marketing, and management of service delivery options.
- B.9.3. Promote occupational therapy by educating other professionals, service providers, consumers, third party payers, regulatory bodies, and the public.

KEY VOCABULARY

Market: All actual or potential buyers of a product, service, or idea; can be considered in its entirety.

Marketing: "The process of planning and executing the conceptions, price, promotion, and distribution of ideas, goods, and services to create exchanges that satisfy individual and organizational objectives" (Bennett, 1995, p. 21).

Promote: To support or actively encourage; further the progress of something.

Social marketing: Techniques of marketing deployed to create positive social change.

If the concept of marketing had been applied to the profession of occupational therapy over 40 years ago, just imagine how much more of a significant role we may be playing in the health and wellness marketplace today! We are the health and wellness profession that assists people in developing the skills they need to participate in everyday life where they live, work, and play. This is our distinct value.

Jacobs K, ed.
*Management and Administration for the OTA:
Leadership and Application Skills* (pp. 57-69).
© 2016 Taylor & Francis Group.

CASE STUDY

Since 2000, the American Occupational Therapy Association (AOTA) has sponsored National School Backpack Awareness Day on the third Wednesday of September. It is actually one of the most successful and sustainable national promotion initiatives for occupational therapy. Joshua is an occupational therapy assistant (OTA) student enrolled in a course on the analysis and adaptation of occupation. His instructor for the course included an assignment where each student is responsible for planning a National School Backpack Awareness Day event in his or her local community. Joshua knows that, as an AOTA member, he can sign up for the AOTA's Backpack Forum on OT Connections at www.otconnections.org. He thinks this will be a good place to network, exchange ideas, and share experiences with other AOTA members participating in National School Backpack Awareness Day.

The need for OTAs, occupational therapists (OTs), and students to fully understand and apply the concepts of marketing and promoting have become even more critical today. Understanding and incorporating marketing and promoting occupational therapy into our daily activities will help us successfully reach the Centennial Vision of the AOTA (AOTA, n.d.) that "occupational therapy is a powerful, widely recognized, science-driven, and evidence-based profession with a globally connected and diverse workforce meeting society's occupational needs."

MARKETING

According to marketer Peter Drucker, "The aim of marketing is to make selling superfluous" (Kotler & Murray, 1975). Marketing consists of meeting people's needs in the most efficient and, therefore, profitable manner (Cromwell, 1984). Kotler and Clarke (1987) defined marketing as "the process of planning and executing the conceptions, price, promotion, and distribution of ideas, goods, and services to create exchanges that satisfy individual and organizational objectives." (Bennett, 1995, p. 21)

Marketing is the wide range of activities involved in making sure that you're continuing to meet the needs of your customers and getting value in return. Marketing can be divided into two types: inbound and outbound. Inbound marketing includes doing market research, analyzing the competition, finding a market niche, and pricing products and services, whereas outbound marketing includes promoting (i.e., advertising, publicity, sales promotion, and personal selling).

MARKETING PLANNING

Successful marketing planning begins with an idea that serves as the framework for all marketing efforts. It is an orientation that makes satisfying the customer's needs the integrating organizational principle. Although the first impulse of the marketing novice is to design a program, such as an early intervention program, and then look for customers (e.g., young children with autism), effective marketing dictates that the process be reversed. You look at the market and listen carefully to potential customers and then design the program to match the needs and desires of these potential customers or in marketing terms, markets.

The main benefits of marketing planning can be summarized as follows (Branch, 1962):

- Encourages systematic thinking ahead
- Leads to better coordination of organizational efforts

- Leads to the development of performance standards for control
- Causes the individual/organization to sharpen its guiding objectives and policies
- Results in better preparedness for sudden developments

The first steps in marketing planning are identifying attractive target markets, selecting target markets and market segments, and developing marketing strategies. Execution of the marketing plan is the second step. It includes carrying out the action programs. The third and final step involves marketing control and requires measuring results, analyzing the causes of poor results, and taking corrective action. Adjustments in the plan, its execution, or both would include corrective actions that could be implemented.

Identifying Attractive Target Markets

Identifying the demands of the market is the first step in marketing. The market is defined as all actual or potential buyers of a product, service, or idea and can be considered in its entirety, such as all referral sources to an early intervention program, or divided into relevant segments according to variables, such as types of professionals (e.g., physicians, special education teachers, nurses). Identifying attractive target markets includes the analysis of marketing opportunities. This analysis consists of the following:

- Self-audit
- Consumer analysis
- Competitive analysis
- Environmental assessment

Self-Audit

A self-audit assesses the strengths, weaknesses, opportunities, and threats (SWOT) of your department and/or specific program. You can even conduct your own self-audit, particularly whenever you are updating your résumé. Factors to be assessed in a SWOT analysis might include the following:

- The reputation of your facility in the community
- The staff and their qualifications, such as certification in any of the specialty certification available through the AOTA
- Physical size of the program
- Location of the program (e.g., school, home, hospital/rehabilitation setting, community-based)
- Convenience of your location to mass transit, highways, and parking
- Type and quality of equipment
- Available budget
- Support from administration

These self-audits assist us in understanding how well or poorly prepared you are to meet the marketplace demands. Ascertaining what you do well and maintaining that product (service) at an optimal level is part of marketing.

Consumer Analysis

It is important to assess the potential consumers of your occupational therapy department's services within your catchment area. An analysis of some of the consumers who might use your products may include clients (individual, group, or population), colleagues (such as physical therapists, athletic trainers, nutritionists, dieticians, and speech-language pathologists), physicians, rehabilitation managers and consultants, other health and rehabilitation professionals, nurses, vocational counselors, special education teachers, attorneys, those in business and industry, administrators, and social workers, among others.

Competitive Analysis

How adequately the needs of the marketplace are being met, what areas are not being served, where duplication and overlap are occurring, and where opportunities for collaboration or joint venture exist can be determined through an analysis of other providers of similar services. One simple way to obtain information is to place your name on the mailing list of facilities/companies providing a similar product line. Reading through newsletters and brochures from the competition can be insightful. You want to learn as much as possible about the providers of similar services so you can be 10% better or 10% different from them.

Environmental Assessment

The changes and trends that may have an impact on occupational therapy services, and perhaps the future of the profession, are comprised by an environmental assessment. These include the following:

- Demographic variables
- Political and regulatory systems
- Cultural environment
- Economic/financial environment
- Psychographics
- Technological developments

Demographic Variables

Demographics include variables such as age, sex, family size, family life cycle, income, occupation, education, religion, race, and nationality. For example, the increasing number of aging Baby Boomers is a demographic trend that is having a significant impact on the demand for occupational therapy services.

Political and Regulatory Systems

Both political and regulatory systems have an impact on occupational therapy services. The Patient Protection and Affordable Care Act of 2010 (P.L. 111–148), Physician Fee Schedule Final Rule for CY 2013, Multiple Procedure Payment Reduction, and the Americans with Disabilities Act Amendments Act of 2008 (P.L. 110-325, ADAAA; see Chapter 1) are some examples that impact occupational therapy. You can keep up-to-date on political and regulatory issues as a member of AOTA by going to its website at www.aota.org.

Cultural Environment

Culture is a force that affects behaviors, values, perceptions, and the preferences of clients/markets. The United States is becoming a more multicultural society, and it is imperative that occupational therapy practitioners and students develop an understanding of and sensitivity to the cultural profiles of their clients. Being bilingual can be most beneficial and may be the variable that assists in making your services even more marketable.

Economic/Financial Environment

An analysis of the economic/financial environment is important because it allows occupational therapy practitioners and students to target occupational therapy services to trends.

Psychographics

Psychographics are lifestyle characteristics about clients/markets that provide information on activities, interests, and opinions of these individuals, groups, or populations. Understanding the psychographic profile of your clients helps provide information to assist in marketing and promoting products and services to them.

Technological Developments

The technology arena is greatly advancing and has an almost daily effect on the type of assessment and intervention used by occupational therapy practitioners. Specifically, information technology allows for information to be exchanged in a more efficient manner.

SELECTING TARGET MARKETS AND MARKET SEGMENTS

Once the market analysis is completed, there are three steps in target marketing. Market segmentation refers to the act of dividing a market into distinct groups of buyers who might require separate products and marketing mixes. For example, physicians can be segmented into pediatricians or neurologists, and health and rehabilitation professionals can be segmented into occupational therapy practitioners, speech pathologists, physical therapists, and athletic trainers. Market targeting is the act of evaluating and selecting one or more of the markets to enter. An example of this is targeting pediatricians as the main referral source for an early intervention program.

DEVELOPING MARKETING STRATEGIES

Product positioning is the act of formulating a competitive position for the product and a detailed marketing mix. Developing marketing strategies includes the development of objectives for each identified target market and their implementation. The 4 Ps—product, place, price, and promotion—are the strategies that can be used to influence the demand for a product (Kotler, 1983a; McCarthy, 1999). Here is how each of these "Ps" is used in the marketing mix.

Product

Simply stated, what we do as occupational therapy practitioners is our product. That is, we help individuals, groups, and populations through engagement in occupation. We are a health and wellness profession that assists people in developing the skills they need to participate in everyday life where they live, work, and play. This is our distinct value. Ideally, we want to offer our market(s) a product line of services—a variety of products associated with one another by an overall theme.

Place

OT services can be provided in a variety of settings almost anywhere. For example, using telehealth technologies and complying with licensure laws, you could provide early intervention to a child in another state without even leaving your home office (see Chapter 1). You might have a "business on the go," where you go to your clients and do not have a physical location other than your vehicle, which transports you and your equipment to your clients. However, some typical locations for our services include:

- Free-standing facilities located in professional buildings, industrial parks, and shopping centers
- Free-standing facilities affiliated with outpatient service departments, rehabilitation centers, or hospitals
- Comprehensive rehabilitation or acute-care facility/program/hospital
- Worksite programs provided by a company to serve the needs of a specific business or industry
- Schools
- Skilled nursing facilities
- Sub-acute/transitional care unit
- Independent living facilities
- Assistive living facilities
- Client's home

When analyzing the place aspect of the marketing planning, other variables that should be considered are the hours the program is offered for business. For example, are your services available during hours convenient to your clients or your staff?

Price

The price or fee schedule for occupational therapy services (products) should be based on cost, competitive factors, geographic area, and what the consumer is willing to pay. It is important for the price to be commensurate with perceived value (Miller & Jacobs, 2007).

Promotion

Promotion is the vehicle of communicating information to your markets (clients) about the product's merits, place, and price. Instruments of promotion are advertising, sales promotion, publicity, and personal selling.

Advertising

Advertising involves the use of a paid message presented in a recognized medium and by an identified sponsor, with the purpose of informing, persuading, and reminding. Some advertising vehicles include the following:

- Print ads found in a newspaper, journal, or magazine
- Brochures
- Direct mail
- Broadcast
- Transit
- Billboards
- Quarterly newsletters
- Business cards
- Bumper stickers (Figure 5-1)

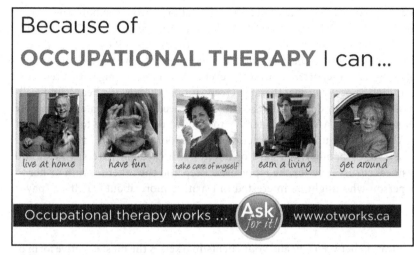

Figure 5-1. The Canadian Association of Occupational Therapists (CAOT) promotional campaign. (Reprinted with permission from the Canadian Association of Occupational Therapists.)

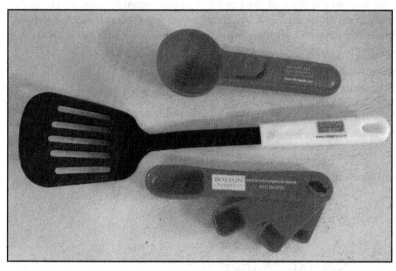

Figure 5-2. Examples of sales promotion items that might be given away at a conference.

Sales Promotion

Sales promotion is the use of a wide variety of short-term incentives to encourage the purchase of or promote a product or service. Some examples of sales promotions are pens, pencils, magnets, tote bags, Post-it notes, and mousepads that you might pick up when going into the exhibit halls at your state conference or the annual AOTA conference. Some examples of sales promotions can be seen in Figure 5-2.

In our case study about AOTA's National School Backpack Awareness Day, Joshua has decided to give out hangtags for backpacks. He will give each child who participates in the backpack weigh-in at a local elementary school a hangtag. The hangtag will promote occupational therapy by having a definition of the profession on the hangtag along with the AOTA's logo and Backpack tag line: Pack it Right! Wear it Light!

Publicity

Publicity is often a relatively underused aspect of promotion in relation to the real contribution it can make (Kotler, 1983b). The most positive aspect of publicity is that it is free. However, you have little control over the placement of it and, thus, it becomes difficult to focus publicity on specific target markets. An example of publicity might be for Joshua, the OTA student in our case study, to contact the local newspaper and television and radio stations through submitting a press release about his planned AOTA's National Backpack Awareness Day event at a local elementary school. He was delighted to find an example of a press release networking on the Backpack Forum on the AOTA OT Connections (Figure 5-3). If the media finds the event newsworthy and are not understaffed, they will often send a reporter to cover the event. When interacting with a reporter, be sure to share the definition of occupational therapy: Occupational therapy is a health and wellness profession that assists people in developing the skills they need to participate in everyday life where they live, work, and play. Another strategy is to offer to be a resource to them about occupational therapy. Always follow up your interaction with a reporter by sending a thank you via an e-mail, telephone call, or handwritten card or letter. With cards or letters, you should always include two business cards—one for the reporter to keep and the other for him or her to pass along to another person who might be interested in learning more about OT. It's a "pay it forward" approach.

Personal Selling

Face-to-face communication between you and your clients/markets is the most effective form of promotion, the most expensive, and the method used most by occupational therapy practitioners (Jacobs, 1987). Word-of-mouth recommendations by clients who have received or are receiving occupational therapy services is a powerful promotion strategy. Other successful personal selling methods include the following:

- Exhibiting at various conferences
- Developing a free speakers' bureau
- Presenting in-service training to physicians and health and wellness professionals
- Presenting continuing education workshops
- Lecturing
- Attending professional meetings for various organizations
- Holding an open house
- Holding continuing education seminars for referral sources

SOCIAL MARKETING

The AOTA National School Backpack Awareness Day that Joshua is participating in is a good example of social marketing, which uses the techniques of marketing to effect positive social change. Other such examples are the non-profit, Rebuilding Together, which provides low-income homeowners with rebuilding services, and CarFit, which is a program that assists older drivers with safety and mobility.

Social Media

Social media, which include social networking sites, such as Facebook and LinkedIn, micro-blogs, such as Twitter, and content communities, such as YouTube, may be used for effective marketing. In our case study, Joshua is using Facebook to promote the AOTA National School Backpack Awareness Day event at the local elementary school. Joshua is very careful to avoid using professional jargon in his postings on Facebook and when discussing occupational therapy with the elementary students and their teachers.

News Release

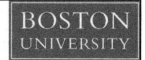

Boston University College of Health
& Rehabilitation Sciences: Sargent College

FOR IMMEDIATE RELEASE:
CONTACT: Stephanie Rotondo, (617) 353-7476, rotondos@bu.edu

BU SARGENT COLLEGE ERGONOMIC EXPERT ASKS STUDENTS 'WHAT'S IN YOUR BACKPACK?'

BU Professor Raises Awareness about Health Risks of Overloaded Backpacks

(Boston) — In honor of National School Backpack Awareness Day™ on Wednesday, September 17, 2014, Dr. Karen Jacobs, a Boston University Sargent College occupational therapy professor and former president of the American Occupational Therapy Association (AOTA), will be conducting "weigh-ins" at a Boston area school to ensure that the weight of kids' backpacks exceeds no more than 10% of their body weight. This annual event helps educate children, parents, school administrators, teachers, and the community about the serious health problems associated with wearing a backpack incorrectly.

Jacobs and 62 graduate OT students from Boston University College of Health and Rehabilitation Sciences: Sargent College will be at the Jackson Mann School in Brighton, MA from 10 a.m. to 11:30 p.m. on September 17. Jacobs and her graduate students will weigh the backpacks of elementary school students and offer guidance on the best way to wear a backpack. Carrying too much weight in a pack or wearing it the wrong way can lead to aching back and shoulders, weakened muscles, and stooped posture.

"More than 72 million American school children will be wearing a backpack to and from school every day this academic year. And as OTs, we're concerned about the increasingly serious problem posed by improper school backpack use," says Jacobs. "We risk doing long-term damage to our kids' growing bodies by remaining silent on this public health issue."

Jacobs advises minimizing long-term health problems by loading the heaviest items closest to the child's back and arranging books and materials so they won't slide around in the backpack.

Figure 5-3. Example of a news release/press release. (*continued*)

Jacobs supports the effectiveness of backpack education. In a study, almost 8 out of 10 middle school children who had been educated on backpack safety subsequently changed how they loaded their backpacks and ultimately reported less pain and strain in their backs, necks, and shoulders.

Dr. Karen Jacobs is a sought after ergonomics expert who champions backpack and computer safety for children and teens. She conducts research, writes, and speaks about these topics regularly. She is a clinical professor of occupational therapy at Boston University College of Health and Rehabilitation Sciences: Sargent College, the former president of the American Occupational Therapy Association (AOTA), and a recent winner of the Eleanor Clarke Slagle Award, the highest academic honor given by the AOTA. Jacobs is the recent author of the children's book *How Full Is Sophia's Backpack*, which integrates tips on proper backpack usage into its imaginative story.

Boston University **College of Health and Rehabilitation Sciences: Sargent College** is an institution of higher education which fosters critical and innovative thinking to best serve the health care needs of society through academics, research, and clinical practice. As reported by *U.S. News and World Report*, its graduate programs in Speech-Language Pathology and Physical Therapy are ranked in the top 8% of all programs, while Occupational Therapy is #2 in the nation. For more information and to learn about degree programs in occupational therapy, physical therapy, speech, language, and hearing sciences, health science, athletic training, human physiology, behavior and health, and nutrition, visit bu.edu/sargent.

Founded in 1839, Boston University is an internationally recognized private research university with more than 30,000 students participating in undergraduate, graduate, and professional programs. BU consists of 16 colleges and schools, along with a number of multi-disciplinary centers and institutes which are central to the school's research and teaching mission.

Figure 5-3 (continued). Example of a news release/press release.

EXECUTION OF THE MARKETING PLAN

Once you have selected your target market, develop a specific marketing mix (product, price, place, and promotion) for your market that stresses the benefits and distinct value of your occupational therapy products. When executing action programs, a timeline should be delineated, such as a 12-month period, to measure whether objectives and goals are being met. The action plan should be dynamic and able to be changed throughout the year as new opportunities and problems arise. Ideally, actions should be assigned to specific individuals who are given exact completion dates.

Marketing Control

Marketing is an area where rapid obsolescence of objectives, policies, strategies, and programs is a constant possibility (Kotler & Clarke, 1984). Marketing control attempts to circumvent this dilemma and assists in maximizing the probability that a product will achieve its short- and long-term objectives. It is important to measure program results, diagnose these results, and take corrective action, if necessary. There are three types of marketing control (Kotler & Clarke, 1984):

1. Annual plan control consists of the steps used during the year to monitor and correct deviations from the marketing plan to ensure that annual sales and profit goals are being achieved.

2. Profitability control refers to the efforts used to determine the actual profit or loss of different marketing entities such as the products (services) or market segments.

3. Strategic control is a systematic evaluation of the organization's market performance in relation to the current and forecasted marketing environment.

CONCLUSION

A bright future can be a certainty for occupational therapy practitioners and students who are prepared to accept the reality of today and tomorrow's health and wellness environment. It will be increasingly competitive with various professions vying for control of limited resources that are increasingly complex, accountable, and increasingly controlled by third party payers and the government.

Occupational therapy practitioners and students' abilities to market and promote their skills and knowledge to those that control the dollars will be an ever-present requirement for success. It will likely make the difference between encroachment by other professions.

We live in a world of limited resources that is technologically complex, economically competitive, and growing more politically accountable with consumer power on the rise. The good news is that this is a world of limitless opportunities for occupational therapy. However, we must work diligently—individually and collectively—to ensure that occupation is recognized as our central construct and to communicate how it shapes and informs our methods and outcomes through infusion in education, research, and practice. We must be aggressive in our support of, and advocacy for, scientific inquiry and pragmatic investigation that build the profession's evidence-based body of knowledge. We must participate in strategic partnerships and interprofessional teams to construct communities where human occupation is recognized as fundamental to quality of life and social participation, as well as central to social, educational, and health care policies in the United States and the global community. We can and will reach this envisioned future. (Jacobs, 2012, p. 652).

SUGGESTED WEBSITES

- Entrepreneur: http://www.entrepreneur.com/marketing
- American Marketing Association: https://www.ama.org/Pages/default.aspx
- Introduction to Marketing free course from the University of Pennsylvania, Wharton: https://www.coursera.org/course/marketing

REVIEW QUESTIONS

1. An individual's lifestyle characteristics are measured by the technique called:
   a. Cognitive analysis
   b. Psychographics
   c. Life cycle analysis
   d. Lifestyle integrative assessment

2. The most common promotional technique used by occupational therapy practitioners is:
   a. Advertising
   b. Personal selling
   c. Sales promotion
   d. Publicity

3. A market is:
   a. All actual or potential buyers of a product, service, or idea
   b. A place
   c. A price
   d. Transactions between the buyer and seller of a product

4. Which of the following statements regarding the benefits of marketing planning is false?
   a. It encourages systematic thinking.
   b. It results in better preparedness for sudden development.
   c. It leads to better coordination of an organization's efforts.
   d. It leads to the development of poorer performance standards for control.

5. The four P's of the marketing mix are:
   a. Price, packaging, place, and promotion
   b. Place, price, promotion, and product
   c. Product, packaging, promotion, and place
   d. Product, procedure, price, and packaging

6. The three-step process for marketing planning and control is:
   a. Planning, execution, and control
   b. Control, execution, and planning
   c. Execution, planning, and control
   d. Planning, control, and execution

7. What is not a type of marketing control?
   a. Annual plan control
   b. Profitability control
   c. Strategic control
   d. Segment marketing control

8. What are the three steps in target marketing?

   a. Market segmentation, market targeting, and product positioning

   b. Market segmentation, market targeting, and price positioning

   c. Product positioning, price targeting, and market segmentation

   d. Market targeting, market pricing, and target placement

9. What does the letter S stand for in a SWOT analysis?

   a. Super

   b. Strength

   c. Strong

   d. Statistics

10. When you go to a conference and a vendor gives you a magnet, it is an example of what kind of promotion?

    a. Publicity

    b. Personal selling

    c. Public relations

    d. Sales promotion

REFERENCES

American Occupational Therapy Association. (n.d.). *The road to the Centennial vision.* Retrieved from http://www. aota.org/ News/Centennial.aspx

Bennett, P. D. (1995) *Dictionary of marketing terms.* Chicago: American Marketing Association.

Branch, M. (1962). *The corporate planning process.* New York: American Management Association.

Jacobs, K. (1987). Marketing occupational therapy. *American Journal of Occupational Therapy, 41*(5), 315-320.

Jacobs, K. (2012). PromOTing occupational therapy: Words, images, and actions (Eleanor Clarke Slagle lecture). *American Journal of Occupational Therapy, 66,* 652-671.

Kotler, P. (1983a). *Principles of marketing* (2nd ed.). Englewood Cliffs, NJ: Prentice Hall.

Kotler, P. (1983b). *Principles of marketing—instructor's manual with cases.* Englewood Cliffs, NJ: Prentice Hall.

Kotler, P., & Clarke, R. (1984). *Marketing management* (5th ed.). Englewood Cliffs, NJ: Prentice Hall.

Kotler, P., & Clarke, R. (1987). *Marketing for health care organizations.* Englewood Cliffs, NJ: Prentice Hall.

Kotler, P., & Murray, M. (1975). Third sector management: The role of marketing. *Public Administration Review, 35*(5), 469.

McCarthy, E. J. (1999). *Basic marketing: A managerial approach* (13th ed.). Homewood, IL: Irwin.

Miller, D., & Jacobs, K. (2007). Economics and marketing of ergonomic services. In K. Jacobs (Ed.), *Ergonomics for therapists.* St. Louis, MO: Elsevier.

6

Documentation and Quality Improvement

Brenda Kennell, BS, MA, OTR/L

ACOTE Standard explored in this chapter:

- Standard B.7.6. Participate in the documentation of ongoing processes for quality improvement and implement program changes as needed to ensure quality of services.

KEY VOCABULARY

Accreditation: The process through which an organization receives "approval" for meeting a specific set of criteria or standards determined by an outside organization. Accreditation organizations include the National Committee for Quality Assurance, the Joint Commission (formerly JCAHO), and ACOTE.

Benchmark: A way for an organization to analyze quality data internally or against data from other organizations that are similar in size, location, and services.

Documentation: Generally refers to the recording in written or electronic form of information regarding the client in occupational therapy. It includes evaluations, plans of care, progress reports, discharge summaries, Individualized Education Plans (IEPs), Medicare recertifications, and other forms.

Quality: How good or bad something is. In health care, this would generally be defined as receiving "the right services, at the right time, and in the right way to achieve the best possible health" (National Quality Forum, 2014).

Jacobs K, ed.
Management and Administration for the OTA:
Leadership and Application Skills (pp 71-90).
© 2016 Taylor & Francis Group.

Quality assurance: A system of determining quality mainly through retrospective scrutiny of records. The system included identifying and counting errors that were deviations from an established standard and determining an action plan to reduce reoccurrence of the errors.

Quality control: Managing quality by focusing on finding defects, rejecting defective products, and determining how to alter processes to produce products with fewer deficits.

Quality improvement: The work that people and the organization are doing to improve health care and the services provided.

Quality measures and performance improvement: Established standards by which current health care practice is measured and a collaborative process aimed at improving the ability of an organization to deliver high-quality services.

Standards: Stated criteria that are used to determine minimal acceptable level of performance.

In health care, there is a saying, "If it is not documented, it did not happen." This is true in every facet of occupational therapy, including quality. Quality and documentation go hand in hand. This chapter will investigate quality improvement and documentation.

WHAT IS QUALITY? HOW DO WE MEASURE IT? WHO CARES? WHY BOTHER?

How do you determine quality? Very often, the quality of an action, idea, or technique is ascertained by the outcome. People assess quality by how well an actual product or process turned out. In education, the teacher grades the student on the paper that is turned in, not on the great idea that the student had but did not write down. Similarly, in occupational therapy practice the accrediting agency, the state licensing board, the OT, the physician, the resource teacher, and the client can only go by what is documented, not by what the clinician thought about or meant to do.

Let us think about performance and quality as a game with players, rules, play, and score (Figure 6-1) The rules provide the structure for the game; this includes the vision, mission, philosophy, goals, and policies of the organization. There cannot be a game without players: the clinicians, staff, clients, and administration. The process of the game comprises the procedures that occur; in occupational therapy, this involves client assessment and intervention. The outcome of the game is the score. Evaluating the outcome, or conducting a play-by-play analysis, tells you whether the outcome was of the desired quality. Did you win, and did you play your best?

Everyone within an occupational therapy department or program can be involved in measuring and monitoring quality. Just as OT practitioners are always informally assessing clients whenever they interact with them, we are always informally assessing quality: "Did that treatment go well? Is that note good enough? Is this project complete?" However, informal assessment is not good enough. There needs to be formal assessment of quality that is measured and documented. Then, the different players—administrators, program directors, surveyors—look at the quality measures to determine whether they are doing well enough and, if not, what needs to change. We will address the role of the occupational therapy assistant (OTA) in data collection and documentation more specifically when we review different types of quality measures, later in the chapter.

WHY ARE WE MONITORING AND MEASURING QUALITY?

The simple answer is to protect everyone. Ensuring that services are of appropriate quality is in the best interest of the clinician, the employer, and the client. Just like there are referees in games

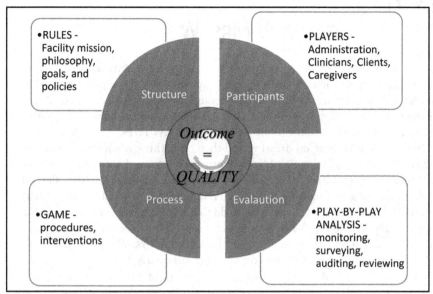

Figure 6-1. The quality game.

•RULES - Facility mission, philosophy, goals, and policies

Structure

•PLAYERS - Administration, Clinicians, Clients, Caregivers

Participants

Outcome = QUALITY

Process

Evalaution

•GAME - procedures, interventions

•PLAY-BY-PLAY ANALYSIS - monitoring, surveying, auditing, reviewing

who ensure that the players and coaches are following the rules and playing safely and the score is accurate, there are various accreditation and governmental agencies involved in monitoring quality and accrediting or licensing health care facilities, companies, and individual providers. Accreditation agencies such as the Joint Commission, previously known as the Joint Commission on Accreditation of Healthcare Organizations (JCAHO), and the Commission on Accreditation of Rehabilitation Facilities (CARF) periodically survey health care facilities and award accreditation. State agencies such as the Department of Health and Human Services are involved in licensing companies such as home health and skilled nursing providers (Scott, 2013). The Accreditation Council for Occupational Therapy Education (ACOTE) is responsible for determining that all OT and OTA educational programs meet the minimum standards of quality set forth in the Accreditation Standards. Individual OT practitioners have to meet the minimum standards of competency set forth by the National Board for Certification of Occupational Therapy (NBCOT) and pass the national certification examination. Each state has a regulatory agency or licensure board that has the authority to grant, as well as suspend or revoke, an OT practitioner's license to practice if it is determined that the quality of the practitioner's service or skills is not current or sufficient (see Chapter 3).

HOW DO WE MONITOR AND MEASURE QUALITY?

The American Occupational Therapy Association's (AOTA) *Occupational Therapy Practice Framework*, third edition (*OTPF*-3) looks at client factors at three levels: person, group, and population. We will examine quality at those same three levels and see the effect on outcome when the documentation is not there or is not supportive. How do we define these three levels?

1. Person: A client, OT practitioner, clinician, caregiver, family member, teacher, physician, case manager, or anyone involved in a client's care.

2. Group: A facility such as a hospital, clinic, or school; an OT department, an OT or OTA educational program.

CASE STUDY #1

TERRY AND MRS. W

Terry is an OTA with 3 years of experience who is working on the inpatient rehab unit. One day, Terry's supervising OT Joanne comes in and says that Mrs. W is going to be discharged to a skilled nursing facility (SNF) instead of going home as she had hoped. When Terry asks why the plan was changed, Joanne says the team was concerned that Mrs. W was not independent in basic activities of daily living (ADLs). "But," says Terry, "she is doing great with her ADLs. We stopped working on dressing and then on bathing when she showed me that she could do it." Joanne scrolls through Mrs. W's progress notes and says, "Terry, it does not say in any of these notes that Mrs. W is independent in these ADLs. It says that she did not want to work on dressing and bathing anymore." Terry replies, "Once she realized that she could dress and bathe herself, she did not want to do that anymore. Why do you think we started working on applying makeup?" Joanne sighs and says, "Terry, we cannot guess why you switched activities. Based on your note, the team thought that Mrs. W was not progressing and was not motivated to keep trying, thus the change to discharge to an SNF."

Terry's incomplete and vague documentation left the quality of Mrs. W's occupational performance up to interpretation. By not specifically stating that Mrs. W had demonstrated independence in dressing and bathing, the decision to change the focus of OT sessions to grooming activities could be seen as a response to lack of progress, interest, or motivation on Mrs. W's part.

CASE STUDY #2

ANDREW AND MIKO

Miko is an OTA with 5 years of experience who is working in an outpatient clinic. Miko applies for a position as a Level II OTA and is turned down. The OT director tells Miko, "I am sorry, Miko. I know all the clients think you are great, but the requirements for the Level II position include competency in the use of physical agent modalities [PAMs]." Miko says, "I demonstrated service competency with all the PAMs last year with my supervising OT Andrew." The director looks again through Miko's personnel record and sighs, "Sorry, Miko. There is no documentation of that. Unfortunately, we cannot ask Andrew, since he left 2 months ago. It is a shame that he did not document it. Maybe you can do the competencies this year and apply for a Level II position next year."

The quality of Miko's skill level as an OTA is unclear. The personnel record indicates that Miko's skill level is still that of a Level I OTA, as there is no evidence of competence in higher-level skills, such as PAMs.

3. Population: Clients with a certain diagnosis, clients at a facility, residents of a facility or location, students in a school, students in an OT or OTA program (AOTA, 2014).

Person

At the person level, quality is generally focused on the outcome of care provided to an OT client and the competence of the OT practitioner. Review Case Studies 1 and 2 and think about whether

Box 6-1
Sample OT SOAP Note in Outpatient Clinic

Name: Chloe Client

Date: 10/26/20xx

Time: 3:00–4:00

- **S:** Client reported that her RUE [right upper extremity] hurt for at least 30 minutes after last therapy session, and that she did not do her home exercises for last 2 days.

- **O:** Client seen for 60 minutes for therapeutic exercise and self-care activities. Client entered therapy with her RUE cradled in her left arm. She was reluctant to start the session, stating, "I'm afraid it's going to hurt more after this." OTA and client discussed her concerns and OTA reiterated that discomfort is to be expected when recovering from surgery. Client verbalized understanding that not doing her HEP [home exercise program] would lead to increased stiffness, which would lead to increased pain.

- **ADLs:** Client reported now being able to brush her teeth by herself, but she continues to struggle with upper and lower body dressing due to decreased strength and ROM [range of movement]. OTA demonstrated alternative technique for donning bra, and client agreed to try that at home.

- **ROM and pain:** Active range of motion (AROM) of the right shoulder external rotation has increased from 15 to 30 degrees in the past 2 weeks. Client is able to complete 10 minutes of continuous mildly resistance UE [upper extremity] activity before needing a rest break. Client was able to demonstrate 3 of 4 exercises on the HEP and was encouraged to try to increase her ROM. Skilled instruction was provided in use of home modalities for pain relief with client returning demonstration.

- **A:** Client's progress has been limited due to post-therapy discomfort, which leads to suspension of home exercises. Client was excited about 15-degree gain of AROM and appeared to be more committed to doing HEP daily. Client is showing increased use of her RUE in ADLs since she has gained AROM.

- **P:** Continue OT 3x week. Discuss with OTR possible use of e-stim for pain relief.

[signed] Pat Practitioner, COTA/L [licensed certified OTA]

there is documentation of the quality of care provided to the client or the competence of the clinician seeking professional advancement.

By *not* documenting what Mrs. W or Miko had accomplished, Terry and Andrew prevented the client and the OTA from achieving their desired, and deserved, outcomes. Even though the OTs knew what Mrs. W and Miko were capable of doing, it wasn't documented and, therefore, did not exist.

Documentation of client intervention is often done in a SOAP (subjective, objective, assessment, and plan) note format (see sample SOAP note, Box 6-1).

Quality in Different Practice Settings

How else can quality and outcome be affected at the person level because of improper or inadequate documentation? It may be something relatively minor, such as an OTA addressing the wrong treatment goal or doing the wrong activity, or it can have dire consequences, such as injury to the client, clinician, or caregiver. Here are several examples from various practice settings:

- The OTA in a pediatric clinic has a client named Tony, who has missed several appointments. The practice manager says that one more missed visit will result in Tony being discharged from therapy. At the end of their session one day, Tony's mother tells the OTA that they will be on vacation the following week and will not attend therapy. The OTA says she will mark it in the schedule book, but she forgets. The following week, the OTA is not working. The substitute OTA notes that Tony missed his appointment, and the receptionist calls Tony's mother and physician to say that Tony is discharged due to attendance issues.

- The OT fieldwork educator at the SNF is very concerned about her OTA student's performance. He tends to use the same activity with several residents, even though their needs and performance levels are very different. It also takes him up to 40 minutes to write a progress note. The OT tells the student her concerns but gives him passing grades on his midterm Fieldwork Performance Evaluation (FWPE). The student does not improve in the remaining 4 weeks, despite her comments and suggestions. The student is shocked at the end of his fieldwork when the OT tells him that he has failed. "I told you that you needed to improve," says the OT. "But you did not write it down on the FWPE as an area in which to improve," says the OTA student. "You said I was at the expected level at midterm. I am writing notes in 20 minutes each now. I thought I was on track to pass. This is not fair!"

- The OT and OTA at the assisted living facility do not adequately document the swallowing precautions and signs of aspiration for the family of a client with dysphagia. The client knows he cannot drink any water because it is a thin liquid, but he drinks the iced tea his family brings from his favorite restaurant. The client silently aspirates and winds up in the hospital with pneumonia.

- The OTA at the industrial rehabilitation program is working with a client who reminds her so much of her favorite uncle. She knows the client is trying his best in therapy, but he has not achieved any of his short-term goals. The OTA worries that Workers' Compensation will force a discharge because of lack of progress and the client will lose his job. The OTA documents more progress than she actually sees from the client. A few days later, the case manager determines that the client is ready for discharge and return to work based on the notes.

- The home health physical therapist (PT) notices that the client is very dizzy after taking her medication, but it wears off in about half an hour. The PT tells the physical therapy assistant, but does not document it in the client's interdisciplinary communication note. The OTA has to change her visit time and winds up at the client's house right after medication time. When she helps the client up to work on kitchen mobility, the client becomes dizzy, leans on the stove to balance herself, and burns her hand.

- The OTA in the hospital notices that a client's brakes are not working very well on his wheelchair. She leaves a note to tell the OT but does not document it in the chart. That evening while a nurse is assisting the client into his wheelchair to go to the bathroom, the brakes do not hold and the wheelchair moves backward. The client and the nurse fall down and are both injured.

- The school OT learns in an IEP meeting that the student is allergic to nickel. She thinks that is not going to be a problem at school, so she does not document it in the OT plan for the OTA. The OTA takes the student into an empty classroom where he can sit at a desk and work on handwriting. He is more fidgety than usual and, at the end of the session, the OTA notices red welts on the student's legs between his shorts and his socks. She tells the teacher when the student returns to his room, and the teacher explains that he cannot sit in the regular chairs because the legs are made of nickel.

- The OT on the gerontology-psychiatric (Gero-Psych) unit receives orders to evaluate a newly admitted client. She remembers this client from an admission 2 years ago, when the client had a very low frustration tolerance, so the OT does not assess the client in this area or document it. She completes the evaluation and writes a treatment plan together with the OTA. The OTA knows that the client is very lonely and bored and has a goal to develop an interest in a leisure activity. The OTA has been crocheting since she was young and decides to try that with the client. The client cannot coordinate the right tension for holding the yarn and has difficulty inserting the hook into the stitch. After a few minutes, she yells, "I cannot do this **** activity" and throws the crochet hook at the OTA. The client refuses OT that afternoon and does not eat her dinner because she is crying.

In these examples, the quality of the care provided by the OT, the OTA, and other clinicians and caregivers may have been adequate and appropriate. However, because of poor or missing documentation, the client, student, or clinician had an adverse outcome (Table 6-1). The road to a better outcome in each of these situations is better documentation.

Think it through:
Think of an experience in your class, fieldwork, or job when your failure to adequately document something resulted in an adverse outcome. Share with your partner and discuss how this outcome could have been prevented.

Group

There are different ways of managing and assessing quality at the group level. Manufacturing and service industries usually perform quality control, which is an ongoing effort to maintain the integrity of their processes and procedures so that there is a reliable outcome. In other words, they want to be sure they are doing things right so the product will be of the appropriate quality. This process includes looking for defects and rejecting defective products before they reach the consumer (Liebler & McConnell, 2008).

The health care industry used to engage in quality assurance, which had a problem-oriented focus. Departments in a hospital would scrutinize medical records to look for errors and deviations from standard practice and expected outcomes. Generally, the focus was on high-risk, high-volume, and problem-prone aspects of care. This was often done retrospectively, and the goal was to show that problems did not occur or occurred at a sufficiently low rate so that the identified performance goal was achieved (Liebler & McConnell, 2008).

The focus in health care and other industries has shifted to one of quality management and performance improvement. Instead of looking back and hoping that things were done well, the focus is on examining processes and performance to prevent errors instead of catching them or fixing them. The bottom line is: Is the process working so that we are achieving our desired outcome? If not, what needs to be changed? Read Case Studies 3 and 4 and determine how the practitioners involved were monitoring quality and whether they documented their findings (Liebler & McConnell, 2008).

TABLE 6-1	
POSSIBLE ADVERSE OUTCOMES DUE TO POOR DOCUMENTATION	
DOCUMENTATION	**POSSIBLE EFFECTS ON QUALITY OF CARE AND CLIENT OUTCOME**
OT evaluation and OT treatment plan/ plan of care	• COTA may work on wrong goals or treatment area. • Scheduled visits may be too few or too frequent. • Client may not receive the correct treatment modalities.
Progress notes	• Clinician may not recognize progress, lack of progress, or barriers to progress. • Client's discharge disposition may be inappropriate to his level of occupational performance or personal choices. • Client's continued treatment may be jeopardized if a third party payer does not see adequate progress or thinks client has already met goals.
Interdisciplinary communication	• Different disciplines may work on the same thing in treatment, which can jeopardize reimbursement. • Disciplines may present conflicting information to the client and/or caregivers. • Disciplines may have conflicts with scheduling, equipment, or meeting with family and caregivers. • Information about safety concerns may not be shared among disciplines.
Client/caregiver education	• Caregivers may be unaware of client's actual abilities and what is realistic to accomplish in therapy. • People may understand a technique or how to use certain tools and equipment when they are with the clinician and then forget when they are home. Clearly written instructions, photographs, and even videos can help prevent problems.
Safety precautions	• Clients, caregivers, and clinicians may be put in jeopardy if they are not all aware of safety precautions related to medication, falls prevention, treatment contraindications, allergies, seizures, swallowing, balance, sensory or perceptual deficits, or cognitive impairment.
DOCUMENTATION	**POSSIBLE EFFECTS ON STUDENT/EMPLOYEE PERFORMANCE AND PROFESSIONAL DEVELOPMENT**
Fieldwork performance evaluation report	• Student continues to perform at subpar level due to lack of constructive feedback. • Student fails fieldwork experience because actual improvement or skill is not documented. • Student passes fieldwork because of lack of documentation of errors, and client or clinician is injured in the future.

(continued)

TABLE 6-1 (CONTINUED)	
POSSIBLE ADVERSE OUTCOMES DUE TO POOR DOCUMENTATION	
DOCUMENTATION	**POSSIBLE EFFECTS ON STUDENT/EMPLOYEE PERFORMANCE AND PROFESSIONAL DEVELOPMENT**
Performance appraisal forms	Employee is unable to maintain employment or advance in position because of a lack of documentation of competency, accomplishments, and achievements.
OTA supervision documentation	Action is taken on license of OT or OTA due to lack of evidence of adequate and appropriate supervision of OTA.
	OTA performs duties or tasks outside of scope of practice or competence because of a lack of documentation.

CASE STUDY #3
ACOTE SURVEY: ELEANOR AND JILL

ACOTE is on campus for a reaccreditation site visit for the OTA program at State Community College. The program director, Eleanor, an OT, and the academic fieldwork coordinator, Jill, an OTA, were both hired in the last 2 years and have never been through a survey. The surveyors ask Eleanor and Jill about the declining pass rate for their graduates. "Oh yes, we noticed that," says Jill. "We are changing our fieldwork courses so the students will be better prepared for their Level II fieldwork and the certification exam." When the surveyors ask to see the syllabus, Jill explains that she knows what she is going to do, but has not yet written it down. "It is not a big deal," she explains. "I am the one who teaches that course, and I know how I need to change it." The same scenario plays out when the surveyors ask for data about recent graduates and their employment. Eleanor says she sees on Facebook when the graduates get jobs, so she has not sent out a formal survey.

Although State Community College has a reputation for being an excellent OTA program with an innovative curriculum and their graduates' pass rate and employment rate are still in the acceptable range, can you conclude that the quality of the program meets ACOTE standards? The surveyors note that there is no evidence that the program is aware of the declining pass rate or has taken any action to address the change. There is no documentation to support the changes they claim to have planned for the fieldwork courses. There is no evidence that the program is monitoring the employment rate of its graduates. There is only the word of the faculty.

Quality Management

Practitioners in an OT department may use all of the previously described methods to monitor the quality of their interventions and their documentation. Quality control is often used when focusing on documentation and timeliness, such as: Are evaluations completed within 24 hours of receipt of order? A quality assurance focus might be on high-risk or problem-prone diagnoses or procedures, such as patients with dysphagia or babies in the neonatal ICU, and set levels of expected performance. This is usually expressed as a percentage (e.g., 90% of lymphedema clients will show reduction in edema $\geq 25\%$). A quality improvement focus often involves multiple

Case Study #4
The Joint Commission Survey: Jerry and Michelle

Everyone at Valley Medical Center is on pins and needles due to the Joint Commission accreditation survey team arriving this morning. The rumor has been spreading that one of the survey team members is really hard on therapy departments. The surveyor comes into the OT staff office, walks up to Jerry and Michelle, and asks Jerry what he thinks about the documentation in the OT department. Does the new electronic medical record system provide opportunity for writing a thorough and meaningful OT progress note? Jerry nods energetically, agreeing that the format allows him to write all that he wants and needs to include. "How do you know the notes are good?" asks the surveyor. Jerry says he "just knows" and the surveyor turns to Michelle. "I understand this facility sees a lot of clients for hip replacements. Do you think there is a difference in the recovery of people who have the anterior approach versus the posterior approach?" Michelle answers that recovery is shorter and better after an anterior approach. "How do you know?" asks the surveyor. Michelle, like Jerry, says she "just knows" that it is better. The surveyor has one last question for the two of them: "Can either of you show any documentation to support what you have said?"

The accreditation surveyor was looking for evidence of the quality of the OT department's treatment and documentation, but neither Jerry nor Michelle were able to provide that. Is the documentation at Valley Medical Center really good? Are the clients who have the anterior approach hip replacement really being discharged sooner and with better outcomes? How can this be demonstrated?

Table 6-2	
Quality Management for Inpatient Therapy Department Treating Clients With Dysphagia	
Quality control	Are reports from modified barium swallow studies (MBSS) completed on a timely basis?
Quality assurance	90% of clients with swallowing difficulty will have an MBSS ordered.
Performance improvement	Clients with swallowing difficulty will have medication reviewed by a pharmacist, signs posted in room by speech-language pathologist, and patient/family education session with OT.

departments and looks especially at the hand-off of clients from one department or staff member to another. Let us look at how all three types of quality management might be utilized by a hospital therapy department that sees a lot of people with swallowing difficulties (Table 6-2)

Typical methods used in quality management involve collection of data to determine if the interventions were of sufficient quality to result in positive client outcomes. Often a percentage goal or benchmark is set so that the data can be compared with a goal or with results from similar facilities. The goal of data collection is not necessarily to demonstrate perfection, but rather to determine where quality is below the desired level and improvement is necessary. The lists below are examples of quality management in a medical practice setting—inpatient, rehabilitation, outpatient, SNF, home health—although similar items could be used in other settings such as school, community, or mental health settings (Figures 6-2 through 6-5).

Date:	8/4/xx	Clinician: Terry Therapist		Med. Rec. #: 278943			
		INDICATOR: Does the chart include evidence of:	**YES**	**NO**	**N/A**	**COMMENTS:**	
Evaluation and Plan of Care		• Client and family involvement in developing the plan of care?	X				
		• Communication with physician?	X				
		• Communication between therapist and assistant in the evaluation?		X			
		• Pain assessment in evaluation?	X				
Progress Notes		• Progress towards goals?	X				
		• Communication with other disciplines?			X	No other disciplines involved	
		• Communication between therapist and assistant in the notes?	X				
		• Client and caregiver education?	X				
		• Pain assessment in notes?		X		Not in 2/8 notes	
		• Re-evaluation completed on a timely basis?	X				
		• Re-certification completed on a timely basis?	X				
Discharge summary		• Discharge summary with reason for discharge?	X				
		• Discharge summary with referrals and follow-up?		X		Client stopped attending without notice	

Figure 6-2. Sample chart audit.

- Performing chart audit and review
  - Charts (possibly with clinician names removed) can be reviewed randomly for presence of specific criteria
  - Criteria can be objective and checked as present or absent, or as subjective where the reviewer must use clinical judgment to determine if the standard was met
  - Objective criteria can include:
    - Evidence of required components, such as total time of visit, pain scale, minutes per Current Procedural Terminology (CPT) billing code (see Chapter 4)
    - Evidence of non-approved abbreviations, incomplete signatures, or illegible entries

DATE	CLINICIAN	MED. REC. #	TOTAL TIME DOCUMENTED		MINUTES PER CPT CODE DOCUMENTED	
7/21	Billie Brown	544896	YES √	NO	YES √	NO
7/22	Betty Black	648721	YES √	NO	YES	NO √
7/23	Bonnie Blue	364981	YES	NO √	YES	NO √
7/24	Bert Beige	648975	YES √	NO	YES √	NO
7/25	Ben Brick	487329	YES √	NO	YES √	NO

Figure 6-3. Sample chart review.

The staff at General Hospital Occupational Therapy Department value your opinion and comments about your therapy experience. Please fill in the name of your therapy practitioners and score each item on the scale indicated below. We appreciate your assistance in our quest to provide the highest quality therapy to all our clients.

Name:_____ Therapy staff:_____ Date:_____

1= Strongly disagree 2=Disagree 3=Neither agree nor disagree 4=Agree 5=Strongly agree	
1. I did not have to wait too long to be seen	1 2 3 4 5
2. The therapy staff cared about me and my concerns	1 2 3 4 5
3. My privacy and confidentiality were protected	1 2 3 4 5
4. The therapy staff explained things clearly	
5. The waiting area was comfortable	1 2 3 4 5
6. The office manager was helpful in setting appointments, explaining my bill, etc.	1 2 3 4 5
7. I have seen improvement since I started my therapy	1 2 3 4 5
8. I would recommend this therapy department to others	1 2 3 4 5
Comments:	

Figure 6-4. Sample client satisfaction survey.

- ○ Subjective criteria can include:
  - ◆ Evidence of client involvement in setting goals
  - ◆ Evidence of communication between OT and OTA
  - ◆ Evidence of client and family education
  - ◆ Evidence of goal achievement
- • Conducting satisfaction surveys
  - ○ Clients can be surveyed during and/or after completion of their full treatment
  - ○ Criteria can include client feelings such as whether clients feel that:
    - ◆ privacy and confidentiality were preserved
    - ◆ they were involved in the treatment planning and goal setting
    - ◆ they are improved after therapy
  - ○ Criteria can include client's perception of staff, such as whether:
    - ◆ the clinician was caring and paid attention to the client
    - ◆ clerical staff was polite and helpful

Med. Rec. #	729483					
Treatment Diagnosis	R CVA					
Admission FIM Feeding	4					
Grooming	4					
Toileting	3					
Dressing-UB	4					
Dressing-LB	3					
Bathing	2					
Discharge FIM Feeding	6					
Grooming	7					
Toileting	6					
Dressing-UB	5					
Dressing-LB	5					
Bathing	4					
Total FIM Gain	13					
LT Goal #1 achieved?	YES					
LT Goal #2 achieved?	YES					
LT Goal #3 achieved?	NO					
LT Goal #4 achieved?	YES					
LT Goal #5 achieved?	YES					
LT Goal #6 achieved?	YES					

Figures 6-5. Sample monitoring client results.

- ○ Criteria can include client opinion of environmental factors such as:
  - ◆ Comfort of reception area
  - ◆ Length of wait time
  - ◆ Parking availability
- ○ Physician satisfaction surveys can also be conducted
- Monitoring client results
  - ○ Data can be compiled to determine whether therapy was effective. This can include whether clients made progress in therapy, as well as considerations of when therapy was terminated for reasons other than lack of progress.
  - ○ Criteria can include:
    - ◆ Comparison of Functional Independence Measurement scores or other measurements from initial and discharge evaluations
    - ◆ Percentage of client long-term goals that were achieved

Performance Improvement

In addition to the client quality measures that reflect effectiveness, performance may be evaluated by other criteria that reflect efficiency and timeliness of performance. The data may be compared with predetermined goals or compared with benchmarks from other departments or institutions. The criteria may be more focused on performance of the clinicians or faculty rather than the outcome for the clients or students.

- Criteria can include the following:
  - ○ Are client evaluations completed in a set time frame (e.g., 24 hours after inpatient referral)?
  - ○ Are student grades posted within the expected time frame?

In addition to collecting clinical data, facilities and departments may also collect data to determine trends. In a medical facility, this could include which physicians are referring clients or how clients heard about the program. In an OT educational setting, this could include counties of residence for applicants to OTA programs or applicants' scores on admission examinations. This

Figure 6-6. Client Satisfaction—August 20xx.

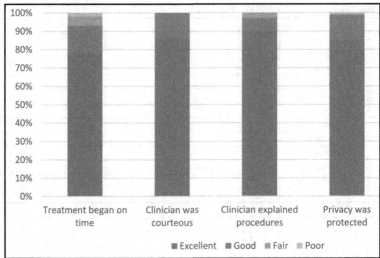

Excellent   Good   Fair   Poor

Figure 6-7. Trending graph sample: How did OTA Student Applicants learn about the program?

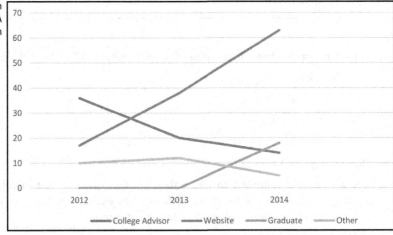

College Advisor   Website   Graduate   Other

information may be compiled and viewed in different forms such as bar graphs, pie charts, and trending graphs (Figures 6-6 through 6-8).

What is the point of collecting all of these data? No practice is perfect and improvement is always needed in the way that assessment, intervention, and interaction are conducted. When the quality data collection reveals less than hoped for results, the next step is to determine how the processes can be improved. The criteria can then continue to be measured to determine whether improvement occurs. To view where the breakdown is occurring, formats such as flowcharts and fishbone diagrams may be used. A flowchart looks at the various steps in a process to see where problems exist and improvement can be made (Figure 6-9). A fishbone diagram considers the equipment, policies, procedures, and people involved in a process to pinpoint where change is needed (Figure 6-10). This is especially helpful in processes that involve multiple departments (American Society for Quality, 2014).

Population

When considering quality at the population level, it is necessary to define the population. How does a population differ from an organization? A population consists of people who reside in a similar location, whether that be a city or a facility such as an assisted living center. A population is also people who share similar characteristics or concerns. This can be clients or service recipients

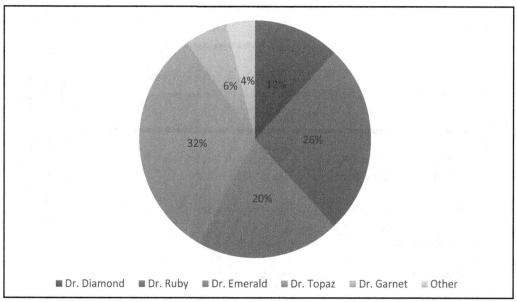

Figure 6-8. Pie chart sample in 20xx.

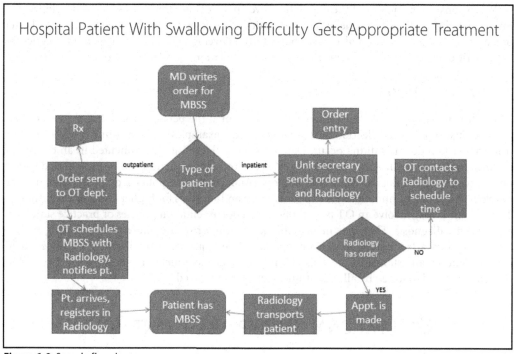

Figure 6-9. Sample flowchart.

with the same or similar diagnoses or presenting conditions or a cohort of students in an OT or OTA educational program. Read Case Studies 5 and 6 and determine the population represented and what they have in common. How is quality being assessed for these populations, and what is the ultimate outcome of these assessments?

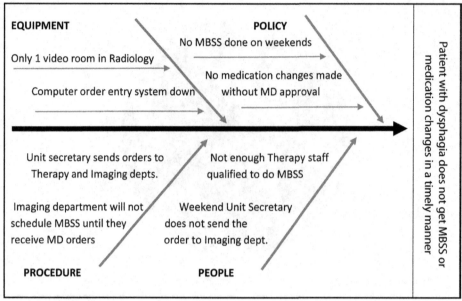

Figure 6-10. Sample fishbone diagram.

When considering quality at the population level, policies and procedures can be developed and implemented that affect everyone in that population. Processes can be changed to achieve a better outcome. This data collection also contributes to the development of evidence-based practice, as OT practitioners can read the literature regarding populations similar to the ones they serve.

Documentation

Quality management and performance improvement at the person, group, and population levels is not just about data collection. Just as we saw in the examples in the beginning of the chapter, if it isn't written down, it didn't occur. Data must be collected and documented in an organized manner so that they can be retrieved and reviewed, and further action can be determined. Based on the review of the data at the group or population level, new policies or procedures may be developed to define minimum levels of performance and set goals for higher levels of performance. These changes may involve an OT practitioner, as in documentation policies or practice standards for a specific diagnosis. They may involve the client, as in providing more privacy during evaluations. They may affect a student, as in change in course sequence or requirements. The new policies, procedures, and standards must also be appropriately documented to ensure that they will be implemented and followed by all practitioners and staff involved.

OCCUPATIONAL THERAPY ASSISTANT ROLE

All members of the OT team are involved in the collection and reporting of data for quality and performance improvement. In a medical or school-based setting, the OTA may be involved in chart audit that requires clinical judgment, reviewing charts of other clinicians and completing a check list. This may include chart review of discharged clients to check for inclusion of pertinent details such as client involvement in goal setting and evidence of client improvement and goal attainment. The OTA may look at data that are completely objective, such as physician referral patterns, accuracy of charges, and timeliness of evaluations and appointments, although this can

CASE STUDY #5
PLEASANT PINES SKILLED NURSING FACILITY

The OT staff at Pleasant Pines Skilled Nursing Facility knows that a significant portion of residents have chronic pain that impedes their occupational performance and general well-being. One of the therapists attends a conference and hears a presentation about the use of diathermy to decrease pain and increase mobility. After discussion at a staff meeting, the OT staff decide to research whether diathermy does provide significant enough pain relief that residents are more able to participate in their therapy sessions and engage in ADLs and preferred leisure activities. The department implements a chronic pain assessment that they administer along with a questionnaire regarding ADL and leisure participation. Over the next 12 months, they collect data during the OT initial and discharge evaluations on all the residents on their caseload who are identified with chronic pain, whether or not they receive orders for diathermy. Data collection is also done at the two sister facilities in the company. After the data collection period, a comparison of the two groups reveals a significant improvement in the residents receiving diathermy. This leads to development of a Chronic Pain protocol. The OT director presents the results to the medical directors and nurse managers of the facilities, and two therapists publish an article in an OT journal.

Data were collected in these facilities for all residents who fit a certain criteria. These data were documented, organized, and reviewed, which led to evidence-based research and publication. Based on review of the data, it was determined that providing a certain modality resulted in improved function and quality of life for a specific population—people with chronic pain who were receiving OT services. Policy changes were implemented, which then made the service available to everyone with that diagnosis. These policy changes would not have been possible based solely on the intuition of one clinician or anecdotal evidence based on one resident. The documentation of the data was crucial to the changes that would then affect the outcome for others in that population.

CASE STUDY #6
CITY COMMUNITY COLLEGE AND TECHNICAL INSTITUTE

Shana is the program director of a new OTA program at City Community College and Technical Institute. She is very excited, but frustrated because the college has not included a medical terminology course in the curriculum or as a general education requirement. During the first 2 years of the program, Shana carefully tracks quiz and project grades in the Foundations and Documentation courses for all the students in the program. She then compares the grades for the students who had medical terminology before entering the OTA program and for those who did an independent study in medical terminology during the Foundations course. She also compares the student satisfaction comments and suggestions on the course evaluation forms. Based on her findings, Shana is able to secure approval to add medical terminology as a prerequisite course for the OTA program.

Tracking grades and satisfaction for all the students in the OTA program is another example of monitoring quality for a population. Baseline quality is being expressed as students who receive passing grades. Baseline, however, represents the minimum level of quality. The program can set benchmarks, as does ACOTE, to establish a desired level of performance that is above the minimum. For example, a program may require students to receive at least a C in all OTA courses, which is the minimum standard, but set a benchmark looking for 80% of the students to receive grades of B or higher in a course. NBCOT sets a minimum score for passing the certification examination, but ACOTE sets a benchmark that requires 80% of graduates to pass the certification exam in the first year after graduation.

also be assigned to nonclinical personnel, such as receptionists, office managers, and rehabilitation technicians. Data that may be reflective of a specific clinician's performance, such as client satisfaction surveys, are usually reviewed and compiled by the department director. School-based settings may involve review of IEPs or student work samples. In an OT or OTA education setting, the ACOTE requires significant amounts of data, as well as data that the institution and/or program may wish to track. Regardless of the setting, the OTA can play a key role in collection and review of data, as well as determination and design of changes to be implemented.

CONCLUSION

In occupational therapy, quality can be described and measured at the person, group, and population levels. OTAs may be involved in determining the type of data to be collected and the method for collecting the data. OTAs may be involved in the actual collection of the data and the review of the data. Just as OTAs and OTs should collaborate on the development of a plan of care for their clients, so should OTAs be involved in determining the plan of action necessary after review of data in their practice setting. Documentation of the findings and the actions is crucial as evidence of the data and the action taken.

SUGGESTED WEBSITES

- Accreditation Council for Occupational Therapy Education: www.aota.org/education-careers/accreditation.aspx
- Agency for Healthcare Research & Quality: www.ahrq.gov
- American Society for Quality: www.asq.org
- Commission on Accreditation of Rehabilitation Facilities: www.carf.org

REVIEW QUESTIONS

1. Which of the following is not primarily concerned with assessing quality?
    a. BBB
    b. CARF
    c. DHHS
    d. JCAHO

2. Which organization sets minimal competency standards for occupational therapy practitioners?
    a. ACOTE
    b. AOTA
    c. NBCOT
    d. OTPF

3. In the OT department, someone reviews charts of clients who have completed their treatment and been discharged. This type of review is called:

    a. Prospective

    b. Retrospective

    c. Antecedent

    d. Postprandial

4. In the OT department, which part of quality management might be assigned to a rehabitation technician?

    a. Deciding whether the entries in the daily notes exhibit evidence of client making progress toward goals

    b. Verifying that the minutes of treatment in the note match the charges entered on the bill

    c. Determining whether the treatment provided was appropriate for the client's condition and stated goals

    d. Reviewing clinician competency for the treatment interventions that were provided to the client

5. In the OT department, who would most likely be reviewing the comments clients wrote about their clinicians?

    a. The OT

    b. The OTA

    c. The rehabilitation technician

    d. The director

6. The rehabilitation director is reviewing the service competency log for the OTA who has been working for 6 months. This is an example of quality management at which level?

    a. Group

    b. Organization

    c. Person

    d. Population

7. The OT department has set a benchmark goal that 95% of clients with carpal tunnel syndrome will have a custom-fit splint fabricated for them. What type of quality measurement is this?

    a. Quality assurance

    b. Quality control

    c. Quality improvement

    d. Quality management

8. An OTA program is collecting data on student scores on admission tests and their grades in OTA courses, to determine that they should raise the minimum score for admission into the program. These data are being collected for the program's:

    a. Performance improvement plan

    b. Strategic plan

    c. Total quality management plan

    d. Yearly statistical review plan

9. Which statement best defines the role of the OTA regarding quality and documentation?

    a. The OTA can tabulate results from quality surveys.

    b. The OTA contributes to chart review only for charts that are anonymous.

    c. The OTA can contribute to the review and determine changes to be made in processes.

    d. The OTA can contribute to chart and data review and can contribute to strategic planning.

10. A team of representatives from nursing, discharge planning, occupational therapy, and physical therapy is meeting to determine why there is so much difficulty getting transition paperwork completed on clients waiting to go to rehabilitation. This committee is working on what type of quality measurement?

    a. Quality assurance

    b. Quality control

    c. Quality improvement

    d. Quality management

REFERENCES

AOTA. (2014a). *Current ACOTE accreditation standards.* Retrieved from http://www.aota.org/en/Education-Careers/Accreditation/StandardsReview.aspx

AOTA. (2014b). Occupational therapy practice framework: Domain and process (3rd ed.). *American Journal of Occupational Therapy, 68,* S1-S48. doi:10.5014/ajot.2014.682006.

American Society for Quality. (2014a). *Fishbone (Ishiwaka) diagram.* Retrieved from http://asq.org/learn-about-quality/cause-analysis-tools/overview/fishbone.html

American Society for Quality. (2014b). *Flowchart.* Retrieved from http://asq.org/learn-about-quality/cause-analysis-tools/overview/flowchart.html

Jacobs, K., & McCormack, G. (Eds). (2011). *The occupational therapy manager* (5th ed.). Bethesda, MD: AOTA Press.

Liebler, J. G., & McConnell, C. R. (2008). *Management principles for health professionals* (5th ed.). Sudbury, MA: Jones & Bartlett Learning.

National Committee for Quality Assurance. (2014). *Essential guide to health care quality.* Retrieved from https://www.ncqa.org/Newsroom/ResourceLibrary/EssentialGuidetoHealthCareQuality.aspx

National Quality Forum. (2014). *Measuring performance.* Retrieved from http://www.qualityforum.org/Measuring_Performance/Measuring_Performance.aspx

Scott, R. W. (2013). *Legal, ethical, and practical aspects of patient care documentation: A Guide for Rehabilitation Professionals* (4th ed.). Burlington, MA: Jones & Bartlett Learning.

Solomon, A., & Jacobs, K. (2003). *Management skills for the occupational therapy assistant.* Thorofare, NJ: SLACK Incorporated.

Supervision

Christi Vicino, MA, OTA/L

ACOTE Standards explored in this chapter:

- B.4.4. Articulate the role of the occupational therapy assistant (OTA) and occupational therapist (OT) in the screening and evaluation process along with the importance of and rationale for supervision and collaborative work between the OTA and OT in that process.

- B.7.3. Identify the systems and structures that create federal and state legislation and regulation and their implications and effects on practice.

- B.7.7. Demonstrate the ability to participate in the development, marketing, and management of service delivery options.

- B.7.9. Identify strategies for effective competency-based legal and ethical supervision of nonprofessional personnel.

- B.9.5. Identify professional responsibilities related to liability issues under current models of service provision.

- B.9.6. Identify personal and professional abilities and competencies as they relate to job responsibilities.

- B.9.7. Identify and appreciate the varied roles of the OTA as a practitioner, educator, and research assistant.

- B.9.8. Identify and explain the need for supervisory roles, responsibilities, and collaborative professional relationships between the OT and the OTA.

Jacobs K, ed.
Management and Administration for the OTA:
Leadership and Application Skills (pp 91-104).
© 2016 Taylor & Francis Group.

KEY VOCABULARY

Service competence: The formally documented process of indicating that the OT has determined that the OTA is competent in specific areas of occupational therapy practice.

Immediate supervision: Occurs when the supervising OT provides face-to-face observation and is within close physical distance of the OTA.

Direct supervision OT: Occurs when the supervising OT is at the site where the OTA is providing occupational therapy services and is within speaking distance of the OTA.

Close supervision: Occurs when the supervising OT provides guidance initially and daily contact is made at the site where the OTA is providing occupational therapy services.

Routine supervision: Occurs when the supervising OT provides guidance initially to the OTA, at the site where the OTA is providing occupational therapy services, periodically reviews all aspects of the services being provided by the OTA no less than every 2 weeks, and provides interim supervision by telephone or through electronic or written methods.

General supervision: Occurs when the supervising OT provides guidance initially to the OTA, periodically reviews all aspects of the services being provided by the OTA no less than every 30 days, and provides interim supervision by telephone or through electronic or written methods.

Entry-level practitioner: An OT or OTA who is beginning to develop the occupational therapy skill set during the first year of practice or the first year of practice in an area of occupational therapy practice that is new to the practitioner.

Intermediate-level practitioner: An OT or OTA who is increasing and beginning to master the occupational therapy skill set.

Advanced practice practitioner: An OT or OTA who is improving the occupational therapy skills and incorporating specialized skills.

This chapter will introduce you to supervision, which will be defined, and levels of supervision will be explored. You will learn the "nuts and bolts" of supervision, the requirements for a formalized supervision plan, and the role that you have in the successful supervision of your career. Being part of a professional team will be discussed; and the collaborative relationship between the OT and the OTA will be discussed.

Let us look at the real life scenario in the case study that demonstrates one example of how an OT would supervise an OTA.

SUPERVISION

Supervision is viewed as a cooperative process in which two or more people participate in a joint effort to establish, maintain, and/or elevate a level of competence and performance. (American Occupational Therapy Association [AOTA], 2014)

Supervision of the OTA is a two-way street. The OT has a legal responsibility to supervise the OTA to demonstrate that the OTA is not operating independently from the OT. In the case study, the OTA clearly is not operating independently. The OT completes the evaluation and meets with the OTA to discuss the results. The OTA completes the Allen cognitive levels assessment at the request of the OT.

"Supervision is based on mutual understanding between the supervisor and the supervisee about each other's competence, experience, education, and credentials" (AOTA, 2014). The services provided by the OTA are an extension of the OT and are being provided under the license of the supervising OT in addition to the OTA's license. The OTA has a legal responsibility to provide

CASE STUDY

The OT evaluated a client who presents with a right total hip replacement. The OT asked the OTA to administer the Allen cognitive levels assessment for which service competency has been documented. The evaluation is analyzed, completed, and signed by the OT. The evaluation data indicate that the client has good memory, judgment, attention span, and safety awareness. The client requires maximum assistance with lower body dressing, lower body bathing, and toileting. The client requires maximum assistance to gather activities of daily living (ADLs) supplies for upper body dressing and bathing, as well as grooming and hygiene tasks. The OTA reviews the evaluation and the OT discusses the evaluation and treatment activities with the OTA. The OTA treats the client on day 1 and documents skilled services provided, including that the patient goals were reviewed with the OT and the client. The OT reviews the OTA's notes for the first two treatments and cosigns each note. After the OTA has been treating the client for two sessions, the client's daughter arrives from out of town for the third OT session. Through conversation with the client's daughter, it becomes apparent that the client's home has a second story and stairs to enter the home. Further discussion with the client and daughter reveals that the client was answering evaluation questions quite clearly but was referencing her previous home and not her current home. The OTA met with the OT to provide an update of the newly obtained information during their morning meeting and the OT updated the client's goals. The OT cosigns the OTA's note for the third treatment session. The OTA integrated new activities to help the client reach the additional goal. The OT cosigns the OTA's documentation for the fourth and fifth treatment sessions and the client is added the following week for one treatment session with the supervising OT.

The following week, the OT sees the client for one treatment session and during the morning meeting with the OTA the following day discusses that the patient is making good progress with the OTA and is scheduled for discharge from OT at the end of the week. The OTA provides the patient with treatment activities to meet the client goals for discharge and documents the progress. The OT cosigns the notes and asks the OTA to put together a home program for the client. The OTA provides training in activities that will provide safe transition to home on the client's last day of treatment along with a discharge note, and the OT completes the discharge paperwork and cosigns the discharge note completed by the OTA. The above case study demonstrates a scenario for an OT's supervision of an OTA. There are over eight examples of the OT supervising the OTA in this case study. As you read the rest of this chapter, you will see references that point out many examples of supervision portrayed in this case study.

skilled services only under the supervision of a licensed OT. Supervision "fosters growth and development, promotes effective utilization of resources, encourages creativity and innovation, and provides education and support to achieve a goal" (AOTA, 2014).

Guidelines for Supervision, Roles, and Responsibilities During the Delivery of Occupational Therapy Services (AOTA, 2014) is the AOTA's most current source regarding supervision and role delineation. AOTA documents are generally reviewed every 5 years. It is advised that you read this document and keep a copy of it at your place of employment for reference in addition to your occupational therapy state licensing board guidelines, requirements, standards, and regulations regarding supervision.

There are various levels of supervision and levels of practice within occupational therapy. The terminology and definitions utilized within the profession can be confusing, as there appears to be no uniform terminology defined across state licensing boards, AOTA, the National Board for Certification in Occupational Therapy (NBCOT), federal regulations, and insurance payers. Table 7-1 should help you understand the levels of supervision and the definitions.

TABLE 7-1
LEVELS OF SUPERVISION IN THE PROFESSION OF OCCUPATIONAL THERAPY

LEVEL	DESCRIPTION OF LEVEL
Supervision	"A cooperative process in which two or more people participate in a joint effort to establish, maintain, and or elevate a level of competence and performance. It is based on mutual understanding between the supervisor and the supervisee about each other's competence, experience, education, and credentials" (AOTA, 2014, p. S16).
Direct supervision	The supervising OT is at the site where the OTA is providing occupational therapy services and is within speaking distance of the OTA.
Immediate supervision	The supervising OT provides face-to-face observation and is within close physical distance of the OTA.
Close supervision	The supervising OT provides guidance initially and daily contact is made at the site where the OTA is providing occupational therapy services.
Routine supervision	The supervising OT provides guidance initially to the OTA at the site where the OTA is providing occupational therapy services, periodically reviews all aspects of the services being provided by the OTA no less than every 2 weeks, and interim supervision is provided by telephone or through electronic or written methods.
General supervision	The supervising OT provides guidance initially to the OTA, periodically reviews all aspects of the services being provided by the OTA no less than every 30 days, and interim supervision is provided by telephone or through electronic or written methods.
Minimal supervision	Supervision is provided on an as-needed basis and can be less than monthly.

Adapted from AOTA [American Occupational Therapy Association]. (1999). Guide for supervision of occupational therapy personnel in the delivery of occupational therapy services. *American Journal of Occupational Therapy, 53(6)*, 592-594; AOTA. (2014). Guidelines for supervision, roles, and responsibilities during the delivery of occupational therapy swervices. *American Journal of Occupational Therapy, 68*(Suppl. 3), S16-S22; and AOTA. (2012). *Occupational therapy assistant supervision requirements: Statutes and regulations.* Retrieved from http://www.aota.org/~/media/Corporate/Files/Practice/OTAs/Supervision/Occupational%20Therapy%20Assistant%20Supervision%20Requirements%20Final%202012.ashx

THE OCCUPATIONAL THERAPY ASSISTANT AS A SUPERVISOR

Taking on supervision roles as an OTA can be a very rewarding experience. The role increases as you move from entry level of practice to advanced level of practice. During the first year of practice, you are considered an entry-level OTA practitioner. While you are beginning to develop your occupational therapy skill set, your supervisor role can include overseeing volunteers and occupational therapy aides, depending on your state licensure requirements.

Intermediate-level practitioners increase and begin to master their occupational skill set after year 1 to approximately 3 years of practice. During this level of practice, the supervisor role can include volunteers, occupational therapy aides, Levels I and II fieldwork OTA students, and Level I fieldwork OT students, depending on the state licensure requirements.

Advanced practice practitioners continue improving their occupational therapy skills and incorporate specialized skills after approximately 3 years of practice with the same supervision roles as the intermediate practice practitioner plus potential management positions depending on the state licensure requirements.

OTAs who wish to move into supervision roles in their careers should begin developing leadership skills (see Chapter 2). Taking on volunteer leadership roles within your state occupational therapy association is a great place to start. For example, participating in the state conference committee is a meaningful volunteer role. Continuing education (CE) opportunities are available on the topics of supervision, leadership, and management within occupational therapy professional organizations, local community organizations, and colleges/universities. Many of these CE opportunities are available online or in a distance education format.

When you are a more advanced practitioner, the supervisory, leadership, and management opportunities are varied. In many states, OTA practitioners are rehab directors, regional managers, recruiters, and entrepreneurs (business owners) (see Chapter 5). OTAs serve on many committees and boards for the different occupational therapy professional organizations at the state and national levels. The key to this path is getting involved as a student and continuing to set objectives to reach your ultimate goal.

PROFESSIONAL ORGANIZATIONS INVOLVING SUPERVISION

As you know, the AOTA is the national occupational therapy professional membership organization. The association's journal, the *American Journal of Occupational Therapy,* contains many written documents that cover supervision, ethics, and role delineation that must be followed as an occupational therapy practitioner. In addition, the AOTA offers training opportunities that include the topics of supervision, management, and leadership. The AOTA website (www.aota.org) provides access to and information about many of these opportunities. In addition, the AOTA website includes the *OTA Leadership Development Toolkit, AOTA Leadership Opportunities for OTAs,* the *Fieldwork Educator Certification Program,* and the *Leadership and Volunteer Opportunities Guide.*

The NBCOT is the organization in charge of the certification process and initial testing for occupational therapy practitioners. It has written the *NBCOT Professional Practice Standards for COTA,* which contains practice domains and codes of professional conduct, supervision, and documentation. There are also leadership opportunities available through NBCOT for OTAs.

Medical insurance companies are the agencies that review the documentation provided for occupational therapy services and provide reimbursement for the skilled occupational therapy services. Documentation must reflect that the skilled services provided by the OTA are under the supervision of the OT with the use of a cosignatures, choice of words when indicating portions of evaluation and assessment completed by the OTA, and frequency of documentation provided by the OT indicating participation in the services provided to the client. The case study at the beginning of this chapter describes the OT reviewing the notes of the OTA and cosigning each note, demonstrating one form of supervision.

Individual occupational therapy state licensing agencies are in charge of issuing licenses for the practice of occupational therapy at the state level. These agencies establish legislation that includes the occupational therapy practice act, administrative code rules, and regulations that also include the state code of regulations and statutes. There are positions on many state licensing boards for OTAs.

In addition to the above organizations, each state has a professional occupational therapy organization that offers CE and leadership opportunities and advocacy.

DOCUMENTS THAT PLAY A ROLE IN SUPERVISION

Every occupational therapy practitioner should be familiar with the AOTA official documents. These documents are available in PDF format on the AOTA website (www.aota.org). For the purpose of this chapter, the documents that guide practice, supervision, and ethics are most important. These include the *Occupational Therapy Code of Ethics and Ethical Standards* (AOTA, 2010); the 2014 *Enforcement Procedures for the OT Code of Ethics and Standards, Occupational Therapy Practice Framework: Domain and Process, Third Edition*; the 2013 *Guidelines for Documentation of Occupational Therapy; Guidelines for Supervision, Roles, and Responsibilities During the Delivery of Occupational Therapy Services* (AOTA, 2014); the 2010 revised *Standards of Continuing Competence*; and the 2010 *Standards of Practice for Occupational Therapy*.

The *NBCOT Code of Ethics* and *NBCOT Professional Practice Standards* for certified OTAs (COTAs) are also important documents to be aware of and are available at www.nbcot.org.

In addition to the previously listed documents, your state occupational therapy licensing board's rules, regulations, guidelines, and policies are vital to your career in occupational therapy and should be reviewed.

SUPERVISION NUTS AND BOLTS

Before intervention begins, the OTA must verify that supervision is available by a currently licensed OT that meets the level of experience required according to state regulations for the OTA. The OT and OTA should discuss any concerns regarding the client's status and planned interventions as needed. In the case study at the beginning of this chapter, the OT took time to meet with the OTA to discuss the evaluation results and intervention ideas, demonstrating another form of supervision.

The OTA must demonstrate service competence on higher-level skills that may be utilized in the intervention. In the case study at the beginning of this chapter, the OTA was asked to complete the Allen cognitive levels assessment portion of the evaluation.

During intervention, the OTA should not perform activities that are not within the scope of practice for an OTA. The OTA should not perform advanced skill activities that service competence was not established with the supervising OT.

After intervention, the OTA properly documents the session and signs appropriately. The OTA should always verify that notes are being cosigned according to corporate policy and state and national supervision requirements. The OTA should also verify that weekly progress notes are being completed by the appropriate individuals within the proper time frame according to state and national requirements.

It is imperative that occupational therapy personnel verify that the supervisor and the supervisee are licensed in states requiring a license to practice occupational therapy. There are some state licensing boards that require the OT and OTA to complete supervision forms indicating the name of the OTA supervisee and the OT supervisor. These states also require a change-in-supervision form to be completed whenever the supervisory relationship changes individuals. Maine and Arkansas are two states that require the filing of supervision forms with the state occupational therapy licensing board.

Supervision ratios are also an important factor to monitor. The number of OTAs that one OT may supervise varies from state to state. An example of very specific requirements can be seen on the Oklahoma Medical Board's webpage "Notice of New Rules" under the Occupational Therapist section, which regulates that an OT "will not sign the Form #5, Verification of Supervision, to be the direct clinical supervisor for more than a total of four occupational therapy assistants or applicants for licensure regardless of the type of professional licensure or level of training."

SERVICE COMPETENCE

Service competence is the formally documented process of indicating that the OT has determined that the OTA is competent in specific areas of occupational therapy practice. When the OTA consistently demonstrates that his or her results on a specific portion of a standardized test have the same results as the OT giving the same standardized test, then the OT can document that the OTA is service competent in that specific portion of that standardized test, if allowed by state regulations. The OT also formally documents service competence after observing various treatment sessions that the OTA competently performs. Service competence was showcased in the case study at the beginning of this chapter when the OT asked the OTA to complete the Allen cognitive levels assessment portion of the evaluation. The OTA had documented service competence in this area. Maintaining a log that demonstrates service competency training and results is another example of supervision.

The OT documenting service competence is an important part of this relationship that allows the collaboration to be seamless. The OT must truly understand the OTA's abilities, and the OTA must truly respect the OT's depth of knowledge. It is this trust in competency that allows each team member to help the client live and experience the most independent life possible in all aspects and roles. That sense of achievement for all involved takes the whole team. The team achievement starts with the OT and the OTA, but it involves all of the members mentioned in this chapter.

The realization that you are successful, accomplished, and able to help others reach their full potential is an amazing feeling that team members share when they are working collaboratively. Think about any sports team you have watched during a winning season and consider how many games the team played and won to get to that high point. Consider the communication that occurred among the players, coaches, and fans; and consider the support that each player, coach, and fan contributed to the overall success of the season.

What does this scenario have to do with occupational therapy? You will be part of a professional team! Depending on where you are working, such as in a skilled nursing facility or rehabilitation facility, this team may be known as the medical team that incorporates all the rehabilitation professionals and medical professionals. In the case of a school system, the team may consist of education professionals, such as teachers, a guidance counselor, or a speech-language pathologist (SLP), as well as rehabilitation professionals.

This team can be a winning team that assists clients (individuals, groups, and populations) in reaching their full potential if each player understands his or her role. Clear communication and working together help to keep the client's goals in mind. One of the keys for a winning team is the collaboration between the OTA and the OT. The second key to a winning team is for you to understand how and when to interact with the other professions.

THE MEDICAL REHABILITATION TEAM

Let's start by discussing the roles of each of the players on your rehabilitation team.

We will begin with the administrator, who sets the tone for your work environment or work culture. The philosophy of leadership (see Chapter 2) that the administrator operates with flows through to the director of each department down to the employees. A facility that requires all staff to respond to any call light that is on, identify the client's needs, obtain appropriate assistance, and follow up with the client to make sure that needs are met has a different administrative expectation than a facility that requires only nursing staff to respond to call lights. A facility that requires all staff to participate in passing lunch trays to clients creates a sense of group responsibility compared with a facility where the nursing assistants pass trays. When you see a maintenance worker pick up a lap blanket that is on the floor stuck under a wheelchair and replace it on a client's lap while addressing the client by name, a sense of family and caring is noted. These actions set a tone that is communicated to the clients, students, families, and caregivers the moment they enter the building. The OTA will interact with the administrator in several ways. In some facilities, the administrator attends case conferences, holds monthly facility meetings, makes department rounds, or makes a point of meeting with staff on a regular basis.

The next important team member is the director of rehabilitation. This is the person who is in charge of the rehabilitation aspect of the team and could be an OT, a physical therapist (PT), an SLP, an OTA, or a physical therapist assistant (PTA). It is common to see an OTA or PTA in this role, but be aware that PTAs have different regulations to follow than OTAs regarding administrative roles. Check your state licensing board practice act and state code of regulations for this information (see Chapter 3).

The director of rehabilitation is also in charge of nonprofessional occupational therapy personnel such as OT aides or rehab aides. It is important to remember that "[a]ides do not provide skilled occupational therapy services. An aide is trained by an OT or an OTA to perform specifically delegated tasks" (AOTA, 1999). If the services performed by the aide are considered routine, he or she should not be billed as skilled occupational therapy service. An aide requires continuous direct supervision when performing the delegated tasks. Aides can be utilized for activities such as data entry, filing, ordering supplies, stocking supplies, and disinfecting equipment and rehab space. Always check with your state licensing board for regulations regarding the use of aides. Check your state licensing board practice act and state code of regulations for this information, as the regulations vary from state to state.

The OT supervisor is the OT you are working with in the care of a specific client. Depending on the setting and its organizational makeup, an OTA may have more than one supervising OT.

The director of nursing is a registered nurse (RN) who is in charge of the nursing team. This team might include an RN, a licensed vocational nurse (LVN), and certified nursing assistant (CNA) staff. The restorative nursing assistant (RNA) programming is often shared between nursing and rehab. The OTA interacts with nursing staff throughout the workday. Examples include asking questions regarding a client's status and asking for help with a client you need to transfer whose wound dressing is not adhered. You may need to convey information that you have observed during a treatment session.

The social services director is a licensed social worker who makes sure the emotional and social needs of clients are met according to specific state laws. The OTA may need to make a referral to social service after speaking with the OT and the client and his/her family.

A durable medical equipment (DME) representative comes from a DME company that sells, or in some instances rents, hospital equipment and medical supplies that clients can utilize in their home environment. Some examples are oxygen equipment, wheelchairs, hospital beds, bathtub lifts, raised toilet seats, and ramps. Insurance may cover some of these items. The OTA may interact with the DME representative to obtain a piece of equipment that the OT and OTA have determined a client will need for safe discharge home.

Orthotics and prosthetics professionals evaluate clients for artificial limbs and orthopedic braces. They then fabricate the device and provide custom fitting on the client. The OTA may need to contact the orthotics and prosthetics company regarding modifications that the OT and OTA have determined are needed for client comfort or increased function.

An activity director is generally a person who has passed a state-approved activity training program, a recreation therapist, an OT, or an OTA. The activity director is responsible for providing activity programming at the facility, completing interest screens, tracking attendance, and documenting participation. The activity director may ask the occupational therapy personnel to help increase a client's independence for a particular activity. The activity director may contact occupational therapy to share an observation that might be helpful during client rehabilitation sessions.

Dietary services includes the cooks, servers, and dietician in the facility, who all aid in making sure clients receive the proper nutritional intake to meet their physical and psychological needs. OT personnel are often with clients during mealtime and may need to clarify something with the dietary services department. When the OTA enters the client's room for a therapy session after mealtime, glancing at the bedside table with the meal tray is a habit that becomes integrated into the OTA routine. Therapeutic connections with clients can often be made by discussing their meals with them. A discussion about not receiving the kosher meal requested or the type of egg desired can trigger the OTA to discuss it with dietary services or make a trip to the kitchen for verification and substitution. Establishing a good relationship with the kitchen staff and dietician is very important to help clients reach their dietary intake goals for good participation in treatment sessions.

Laundry gathers soiled linens, towels, and garments in the facility. Laundry is also responsible for delivering the cleaned garments, towels, and linens. OT personnel oftentimes are working on dressing with clients and need to go to the laundry to look for a specific piece of clothing or find loaner or donated items.

Maintenance provides maintenance and cleanliness of the environment and equipment for the facility, and OTs may need to work with maintenance staff with regard to wheelchair maintenance, hospital bed issues, or an issue with rehab equipment.

SCHOOL-BASED TEAM

Occupational therapy personnel also work within the education model that includes the public school system, nonpublic schools, private schools, and private clinics by providing services to support client goals. The education team includes the administrative title of principal–director of special education, who coordinates client services similar to the director of rehabilitation in the medical model and the rehabilitation team, which includes an OT, PT, SLP personnel, teachers, aides, school nurse, academic counselors, a custodian, and lunch personnel.

The school-based model also includes collaborative meetings between the school-based team and parents, who often bring support persons such as attorneys, advocates, caseworkers, social workers, and community service organization representatives.

THE COLLABORATION

"Unity is strength. . . . [W]hen there is teamwork and collaboration, wonderful things can be achieved."

—Mattie Stepanek (2014)

What type of services would a client receive in health care if any provider worked in isolation from all the other service providers? Having a strong collaborative relationship with the OT you work with is important. The ability to have someone with strong foundational knowledge to bounce ideas off of and to reach out to when you feel you have tried everything is essential. Sometimes you need additional information or need to ask for suggestions for additional techniques to help clients better achieve their goals. This interaction is critical to the success of clients in meeting their goals efficiently and effectively. Likewise, in a strong collaborative relationship, the OTA, who often interacts with the client for treatment sessions on a more frequent basis, keeps the OT updated. The OTA informs the OT about clients' progress, or lack thereof, toward goals determined during evaluation so that the OT can check on clients and revise goals as needed. The relationship is dynamic in that ideas and knowledge on diagnoses are exchanged in both directions, from OTA to OT and from OT to OTA, keeping the information flow timely. Two perspectives analyzing a case and seeking evidence-based practice and treatment interventions always benefit the client. In the case study at the beginning of this chapter, the OTA met with the OT to relay new information regarding the patient's home having two stories, allowing for a team discussion regarding discharge planning and goal modification. This is another example of supervision demonstrating that the OTA is not operating independently from the OT and always keeping the OT informed so goals can be modified. The ability to work seamlessly together for the good of the client is a rewarding and meaningful experience. Knowing what information to have prepared for the OT for an evaluation and the OT knowing how to write good goals for carryover to intervention are irreplaceable. The OT and the OTA thinking alike with regard to goals, interventions, discharge planning, and caregiver training and the OT understanding the competency of the OTA are critical.

CONTINUED COMPETENCY

Continued competency is the process of remaining current in all aspects of clinical skills throughout your occupational therapy career. Professional organizations, private providers of face-to-face CE courses, online CE webinars, college coursework, and trade journals are some of the sources for CE opportunities. Many state occupational therapy licensing boards and the NBCOT have specific requirements for professional development units or continuing education units. The *AOTA Occupational Therapy Code of Ethics and Ethics Standards* (AOTA, 2010, p. 3) states, "Occupational therapy personnel shall take responsible steps (e.g., CE, research, supervision, training) and use careful judgment to ensure their own competence and weigh potential for client harm when generally recognized standards do not exist in emerging technology or areas of practice."

MULTIPLE LICENSES AND WORKING WITH OTHER PROFESSIONS

When individuals are practicing occupational therapy, the occupational therapy license they hold is what they are working under. However, OTAs can hold numerous licenses for other areas of practice. For example, an OTA may also hold a massage therapist license. Clients often are not clear on what is massage compared with soft tissue mobilization and other occupational therapy techniques that may appear to be similar to massage. Another example are OTAs who are dual trained as PTAs. Dual trained practitioners need to make their status clear to the client, family, facility personnel, and reimbursement organizations when OT and PT services are being provided. It is very important to not blur the lines of services being provided with the title you are working under. Always be clear what title you are working under, who you are being supervised by, what service you are providing, and how it is to be billed. Regulations and guidelines for state and national agencies should be consulted regarding licensing issues and scope-of-practice issues.

Always be cognizant that you, the OTA, must be supervised by an OT and not by someone in another discipline, even if that be the director of rehab. Your immediate supervisor must be a licensed OT. The OT must have advanced practice certifications in areas required by the state in order for the OTA to provide those same services. For example, California requires advanced practice certification in physical agent modalities that would include interventions such as electrical stimulation, heat and ice application, and ultrasound. An OTA cannot provide these interventions even with years of experience and training if the supervising OT does not have advanced practice certification.

It cannot be emphasized enough that both the OT and the OTA are responsible for knowing and following the supervision requirements at the state and national levels. The OTA is ultimately responsible for making sure that proper supervision is being provided; keeping current on your guiding documents can assist in this endeavor.

ROLES OF THE OTA/ENTREPRENEUR AND SUPERVISION

There are a wide array of areas and roles for the OTA in occupational therapy. An OTA with advanced occupational therapy experience and additional training in areas such as management could secure a position as an OTA program director, an academic fieldwork coordinator, a clinical fieldwork educator, an OTA educator, or a director of rehab. In addition to these positions, an OTA can also pursue positions such as activity director, community educator, life coach, job coach, and entrepreneur.

When working in nontraditional areas or as an entrepreneur, it is very important for the OTA to review state and national guidelines regarding the use of the OTA credential and supervision requirements. Always protect your license and career. The rule of thumb generally has been when using the OTA credential, supervision by an OT is required. In situations where an OT is not on staff, an OT can be contracted or permanently hired to provide the supervision and the evaluation aspect, if applicable. An OTA who starts an occupational therapy business or nontraditional business utilizing the OTA credential and hires an OT on a consultant basis, for permanent employment, or on a contractual basis would be an example of OTA entrepreneurial supervision.

CONCLUSION

Working together with other professionals and maintaining clinical competence is key to providing excellent occupational therapy services. Understanding the supervisory role of the OT and OTA allows for a healthy partnership to flourish. Arming yourself with the up-to-date rules and regulations of corporate, state, and national organizations that affect the profession of occupational therapy enable you to practice within the legal guidelines and ethical expectations of the profession. Together these three concepts can help you to lead a fulfilling and successful career as an OTA.

SUGGESTED WEBSITES

- American Occupational Therapy Association: www.aota.org
- National Board for Certification in Occupational Therapy: www.nbcot.org

REVIEW QUESTIONS

1. The OTA is working with a client on the mat table and the supervising OT is completing a report on a tablet in a chair right next to the mat table while watching the OTA treatment intervention. This is an example of which of the following supervision styles?

    a. Direct

    b. Immediate

    c. Close

    d. Routine

2. The OTA is administering a portion of a standardized assessment to Mrs. Smith and the OT feels that the OTA has been trained well and has proven accuracy in administering this particular portion of the assessment. What term best describes the above scenario?

    a. Entry-level practitioner

    b. Continuing education

    c. Service competence

    d. Advanced service training

3. The supervising OT provides guidance initially to the OTA, periodically reviews all aspects of the services being provided by the OTA no less than every 30 days, and provides interim supervision by telephone or through electronic or written methods. This describes which of the following levels of supervision?

    a. General

    b. Immediate

    c. Close

    d. Minimal

4. Beth, an OTA, has been practicing for 5 years in a pediatric setting and has taken a new position in an acute hospital working in the traumatic brain injury clinic. What level practitioner would Beth be considered at this point?

    a. Advanced practice level

    b. Intermediate level

    c. Entry level

    d. Beginner level

5. Robert has been practicing as an OTA in a skilled nursing facility for approximately 6 years. Robert has progressively added to his occupational therapy skills by taking continuing education courses in assistive technology and stroke rehab. Robert is the person that the rehab department goes to when they need assistive devices to increase a patient's independence. What level of practice best describes Robert?

    a. Advanced practice level

    b. Intermediate level

    c. Entry level

    d. Beginner level

6. What is generally the title of the person who is in charge of the nursing team in a medical facility?

   a. Administrator

   b. Director of nursing

   c. Director of rehabilitation

   d. Social services director

7. This position sets the tone for the entire facility through each department director:

   a. Administrator

   b. Director of nursing

   c. Director of rehabilitation

   d. Social services director

8. Who is mainly responsible for knowing the supervision requirements of the OTA?

   a. Administrator

   b. Director of rehabilitation

   c. OTA

   d. OT

9. Physical therapy and occupational therapy have orders that allow the provision of a hot pack for Mr. Jones's right shoulder. The OT did not write a goal for hot pack application for Mr. Jones, as physical therapy wrote a goal for it. The OTA is asked by the rehab director, who is a physical therapist, to place a hot pack on Mr. Jones's right shoulder. The physical therapist says that it is okay for the OTA to use hot packs because there is an order under physical therapy. Who should the OTA be listening to for direction?

   a. Administrator

   b. Director of rehabilation

   c. OT supervisor

   d. State licensing board

10. What level of supervision is provided on an as-needed basis and may be as little as once every 30 days?

   a. Close supervision

   b. Advanced level supervision

   c. Minimal supervision

   d. General supervision

REFERENCES

American Occupational Therapy Association. (1999). Guide for supervision of occupational therapy personnel in the delivery of occupational therapy services. *American Journal of Occupational Therapy, 53*(6), 592-594.

American Occupational Therapy Association. (2010). Occupational therapy code of ethics and ethics standards (2010). *American Journal of Occupational Therapy, 64*(Suppl. 6), 17-26.

American Occupational Therapy Association. (2014). Guidelines for supervision, roles, and responsibilities during the delivery of occupational therapy services. *American Journal of Occupational Therapy, 68*(Suppl. 3), S16-S22.

Arkansas State Medical Board. (2014). *Arkansas medical practices acts and regulations.* Retrieved from www.armedicalboard.org/forms.aspx

National Board for Certification in Occupational Therapy. (2014). *NBCOT professional practice standards for COTA*. Retrieved from http://www.nbcot.org/practice-standards

Oklahoma Medical Board. (2012). *Notice of new rules*. Retrieved from www.okmedicalboard.org/occupational_therapists/download/667/Notice+of+New+OT+Rules.pdf

State of Maine Professional & Financial Regulation. *Board of occupational therapy practice laws & rules*. Retrieved from www.maine.gov/pfr/professionallicensing/professions/laws.html

Stepanek, Mattie. (2014). 500 fortunes, prayers, and quotes kept on small slips of paper in mattie's pocket used at speaking engagements per Dr. Jeni Stepanek from www.MattieOnline.com on June 25.

8

Fieldwork

Julie Ann Nastasi, ScD, OTD, OTR/L, SCLV, FAOTA

ACOTE Standard explored in this chapter:
- B.7.8. Describe the ongoing professional responsibility for providing fieldwork education and the criteria for becoming a fieldwork educator.

KEY VOCABULARY

Fieldwork coordinator: A faculty member responsible for overseeing student fieldwork placements.

Fieldwork supervisor: An occupational therapy practitioner who provides supervision to students during fieldwork placements.

Fieldwork site: The location where students complete Level I and Level II fieldwork placements.

Level I fieldwork: Introduces students to the fieldwork experience and different practice settings.

Level II fieldwork: Transitions students to the role of entry-level practitioners in the specific practice settings.

INTRODUCTION

Fieldwork education is an essential component of occupational therapy education. Occupational therapy students need to pass all required Level I and Level II fieldwork placements to graduate from an accredited occupational therapy education program, and be eligible to sit for the national

Jacobs K, ed.
Management and Administration for the OTA:
Leadership and Application Skills (pp 105-115).
© 2016 Taylor & Francis Group.

CASE STUDY

John, an occupational therapy assistant (OTA) student, will be completing his first Level II fieldwork placement in a skilled nursing facility. John successfully completed his Level I fieldwork placements and his academic work. After successfully completing his first Level II fieldwork placement, John will complete a second Level II fieldwork placement in a different setting. John is excited to start his Level II fieldwork placements. Throughout the chapter, you will follow John on his fieldwork placement.

board certification examination (ACOTE, 2011; NBCOT, 2009). Occupational therapy relies on fieldwork supervisors consisting of OTs and OTAs, who work in collaboration with fieldwork coordinators to train and evaluate students to meet the minimal standards for entry-level practice. OTAs play a vital role in fieldwork supervision while working under the supervision of an OT (ACOTE, 2011) (see Chapter 7). Occupational therapy practitioners have a professional responsibility to ensure the future of the profession through fieldwork education. Roles, criteria, and components of fieldwork education will be explored in this chapter.

OCCUPATIONAL THERAPY EDUCATION PROGRAMS

Occupational therapy education programs provide students with the academic portion of their degree. Occupational therapy education programs are responsible for training students to become OTs and OTAs. Each occupational therapy education program creates a mission and vision and embeds them throughout the curriculum design. The fieldwork coordinator for the program is responsible for selecting fieldwork sites that match their respective program's mission and vision.

FIELDWORK COORDINATOR

Each occupational therapy education program must have a fieldwork coordinator (ACOTE, 2011). OTs may serve as fieldwork coordinators for occupational therapy programs. Occupational therapy practitioners (OTs and OTAs) may serve as fieldwork coordinators in OTA education programs. The fieldwork coordinator is responsible for the program's compliance with fieldwork education requirements. In this role, the fieldwork coordinator serves as a liaison between the program and the fieldwork sites. The fieldwork coordinator is responsible for making sure the program's curriculum aligns with the fieldwork sites. In addition, the fieldwork coordinator ensures that students receive proper supervision during their fieldwork placements. The fieldwork coordinator oversees the fieldwork placements and works with the fieldwork supervisors and students in facilitating fieldwork placements.

FIELDWORK SUPERVISOR

The fieldwork supervisor is responsible for supervising occupational therapy students on Level I and Level II fieldwork placements. Both OT and OTA students work under the license of the fieldwork supervisor while completing their fieldwork placement. The fieldwork supervisor is responsible for the student during the fieldwork placement. The supervisor's role is to guide, facilitate, and evaluate the student throughout the placement. Upon completion of the placement, the fieldwork supervisor evaluates whether the student has accomplished the requirements of the fieldwork placement. When the student demonstrates competency, the student passes the fieldwork placement. If the student is not competent, the fieldwork supervisor collaborates with the fieldwork coordinator to prepare the student for another placement. The fieldwork supervisor, fieldwork coordinator, and the student should discuss the areas that the student needs to improve prior to completing a new placement.

Eligibility Requirements for Fieldwork Supervisors

The Accreditation Council for Occupational Therapy Education (ACOTE, 2011) requires that Level II fieldwork supervisors have successfully completed initial certification through the National Board for Certification in Occupational Therapy (NBCOT) and have a minimum of 1 year of practice prior to supervising students on fieldwork placements. Prior to supervising students, occupational therapy practitioners should receive training in fieldwork supervision. Academic programs or fieldwork sites may train fieldwork supervisors. OTs meeting the established criteria may supervise occupational therapy and OTA students on Level I and Level II fieldwork. OTAs meeting the established criteria may supervise OTA students on Level II fieldwork when working under the supervision of an OT (ACOTE, 2011).

ACOTE's requirements for Level I fieldwork are not as strict. Occupational therapy practitioners (OTs and OTAs) may supervise occupational therapy and OTA students on Level I fieldwork, as well as other qualified professionals, including psychologists, physician assistants, teachers, social workers, nurses, and physical therapists (ACOTE, 2011).

STUDENTS

Students must meet all of their academic program's and fieldwork site's requirements prior to starting the fieldwork placement. First, students must complete their academic program's requirements to be eligible for a fieldwork placement. Then, students must complete the fieldwork site's requirements. Occupational therapy education programs may have students complete common fieldwork site requirements at the same time to allow students increased opportunities for placement. Requirements may include, but are not limited to, a physical examination, vaccinations, CPR training, a criminal background check, fingerprinting, drug testing, and individual malpractice insurance. Typically, the fieldwork coordinator or the fieldwork supervisor will notify students of the requirements for specific fieldwork placements. Depending on the site, students may be required to complete orientation through the human resources department of the site prior to starting fieldwork. To avoid delay, students should check and meet requirements prior to starting the fieldwork placement.

Now consider our case study. John successfully completed his Level I fieldwork placements and academic work. Prior to completing his Level I fieldwork placements, John submitted documentation of his physical examination, vaccinations, cardiopulmonary resuscitation (CPR), criminal background check, fingerprinting, and malpractice insurance. The fieldwork coordinator at John's program told him that he would need to maintain current documentation for his physical exam, vaccinations, CPR, criminal background check, fingerprinting, and malpractice insurance. Since John's original physical exam was over a year old, John completed a new physical exam and submitted a copy of the results to the fieldwork coordinator. John identified that he would need to renew his CPR between his first Level II fieldwork placement and his second. John scheduled a renewal course between his Level II fieldwork placements to ensure that he would have current CPR for the second Level II placement. John renewed his malpractice insurance, and his fieldwork sites did not require a new criminal background check or fingerprinting. John's first Level II fieldwork site did require an interview prior to starting fieldwork. John scheduled a time to go in for his interview 1 month prior to starting the placement.

While on fieldwork, students should collaborate and communicate with their assigned fieldwork supervisor(s). In some settings, students may have more than one supervisor; students should report directly to their supervisor(s). If students find they are having problems or challenges at their fieldwork site, they should notify their program's fieldwork coordinator immediately. The fieldwork coordinator will serve as a liaison between the student and the fieldwork site. It is in students' best interests to communicate with their fieldwork coordinator about their fieldwork progress in a timely manner.

FIELDWORK

Fieldwork should provide students "with the opportunity to carry out professional responsibilities under supervision of a qualified occupational therapy practitioner serving as a role model" (ACOTE, 2011, p. 32). Students must successfully complete Level I and Level II fieldwork experiences to graduate from their occupational therapy education program.

Level I Fieldwork

"The goal of Level I fieldwork is to introduce students to the fieldwork experience, to apply knowledge to practice, and to develop understanding of the needs of clients" (ACOTE, 2011, p. 33). During Level I fieldwork, students complete observations in an assigned setting. The setting is typically associated with a particular practice course that students have taken or are currently enrolled in. For example, some programs have students complete Level I fieldwork in physical rehabilitation during or following their physical rehabilitation practice course. The Level I fieldwork experience provides students with the opportunity to observe and participate in clinical practice settings that relate to their coursework. Students may be supervised by occupational therapy practitioners or other qualified professionals, including psychologists, physician assistants, teachers, social workers, nurses, and physical therapists during their Level I fieldwork placement (ACOTE, 2011).

It should be noted that ACOTE now requires students to complete a Level I or a Level II fieldwork experience that "focuses on psychological and social factors that influence engagement in occupation" (ACOTE, 2011, p. 33). Students should expect to complete a Level I or Level II fieldwork placement in a setting that addresses psychological and social factors that affect engagement in occupation (Nastasi, 2014).

Level II Fieldwork

The goal of Level II fieldwork is to develop competent, entry-level, generalist OTs and OTAs (ACOTE, 2011). "Level II fieldwork must be integral to the program's curriculum design and must include an in-depth experience in delivering occupational therapy services to clients, focusing on the application of purposeful and meaningful occupation and research" (ACOTE, 2011, p. 34). OTA students must complete a minimum of 16 weeks of full-time Level II fieldwork, whereas occupational therapy students must complete a minimum of 24 weeks of full-time Level II fieldwork. Typically, students complete the two Level II fieldwork placements in two different practice settings.

Specialty Level II Fieldwork

Upon completion of the two required Level II fieldwork placements, some occupational therapy education programs allow students to complete a third specialty Level II placement. This placement provides students with the opportunity to complete a fieldwork placement in a specialized practice area. Occupational therapy education programs typically send students to common practice settings because they are required to prepare students as entry-level generalists (ACOTE, 2011). Since the third fieldwork placement goes beyond the accreditation requirements, students may opt to complete the third placement to have the opportunity to specialize in a specific practice area (Nastasi, 2012). For example, a student may want to complete a third Level II fieldwork placement in low vision rehabilitation or in a school-based setting.

STEPS FOR A SUCCESSFUL FIELDWORK PLACEMENT

The goal for fieldwork coordinators, fieldwork supervisors, and students is to have students pass their fieldwork placements. Some steps for a successful fieldwork placement include a pre-fieldwork interview, formal orientation, student self-assessment, shared supervision by two fieldwork supervisors, and technological tools to promote independent learning (Nastasi, 2012).

Pre-Interview

Research has found that students benefit from a pre-fieldwork interview (Gutman, McCreedy, & Heisler, 1998; Holloway & Neufeldt, 1995). Fieldwork supervisors should request that students complete an interview prior to their fieldwork placement. The interview provides the students and the fieldwork supervisors with the opportunity to meet and gain a better understanding of the expectations of the placement. The interview also helps to determine whether there will be a good working relationship. Grades are not effective indicators of fieldwork success. Students who communicate with their fieldwork supervisors are more successful on their fieldwork placements (Gutman et al., 1998). When fieldwork supervisors find students interpersonally attractive, the supervisors rate the students more effective (Holloway & Neufeldt, 1995). The personality fit of the fieldwork supervisors and students plays a critical role; therefore, scheduling an interview prior to a fieldwork placement allows the fieldwork supervisors and the students to determine whether there is a good fit, as well as establish strong communication and a good working relationship.

Now consider our case study. John had scheduled an interview with his fieldwork supervisor. John arrived to the interview 15 minutes early, dressed in professional attire. John greeted his fieldwork supervisor by extending his hand and shaking hands with the supervisor. Prior to the interview, John went on the Internet and looked up information about his fieldwork site. John answered his supervisor's questions and asked informed questions about the site. The fieldwork supervisor determined that John would be a good fit for the facility and told John that they would see him in 1 month for his placement.

Formal Orientation

Students also benefit from formal orientation at their fieldwork sites. Formal orientation provides students with an understanding of the expectations of the fieldwork supervisors and the fieldwork site. Kirke, Layton, and Sims (2007) led focus groups and determined that fieldwork supervisors need to have a planned orientation where the requirements of the placement are covered. Students benefit when provided with skill requirements, role clarification, and team members' responsibilities for the fieldwork placement (Robertson & Griffiths, 2009). In addition, students benefit from a structured experience (Kleiser & Cox, 2008). Formal orientation provides a way to communicate to students the expectations of the fieldwork placement and provides key training and resources to support their participation in the fieldwork placement.

Student Self-Assessment

During fieldwork, students need to assess their performance. This helps them to determine whether they are meeting the expectations of their fieldwork supervisors and the site. Students who are aware of their strengths and weaknesses and ask for help perform better than students who are not able to reflect on their practice (Duke, 2004). A common method of self-assessment is journaling (Buchanan, van Niekerk, & Moore, 2001; Maizels et al., 2008). When journaling, students complete a daily log of their fieldwork experiences and then share their writings with their fieldwork supervisors during weekly meetings. The journal provides students with a mechanism to go over their thoughts and concerns during the past week. Students should reread their journals at the end of their fieldwork placements and submit their journals to the program's fieldwork coordinator. The journal provides the students the opportunity to communicate with their fieldwork supervisors and to see their growth over the fieldwork placement.

In addition to journaling, a formal self-assessment should take place at the midterm and final evaluations. These formal self-assessments provide a reflective process to identify areas where the students feel they need to improve prior to completing the placement.

Structure and Validation for Shared Supervision

The field of occupational therapy acknowledges that there is a shortage of fieldwork placements. Both fieldwork coordinators and students know that it is not always easy finding fieldwork placements. Changes in occupational therapy practice have led occupational therapy to examine different models of fieldwork supervision. Many fieldwork sites employ part-time practitioners to cover the sites' caseloads. As a result, students completing fieldwork at those sites would have to have more than one fieldwork supervisor.

Literature supports students having one or two fieldwork supervisors during fieldwork placements (Bonello, 2001; Nolinske, 1995; Thomas et al., 2007). Supervision by two fieldwork supervisors provides opportunities to complete fieldwork in emerging practice settings as well as settings that do not have full-time OTs (Bonello, 2001). A study completed in Australia reported that 96% of participating students completed fieldwork with one or two fieldwork supervisors (Thomas et al., 2007). Placing students with two fieldwork supervisors provides increased opportunities for placement, as well as increased opportunities to learn from the occupational therapy practitioners.

Technological Tools to Promote Independent Learning

Technology provides students with opportunities to learn and collaborate with their fieldwork coordinator during their fieldwork placements. Some students complete fieldwork placements close to their academic programs, while other students return to their hometowns or decide to complete fieldwork at other locations. Web-based instruction allows fieldwork coordinators and students to communicate throughout the fieldwork placement. The fieldwork coordinator may post discussion boards to allow students to share experiences with other students or have specific topics that they want students to post on during their fieldwork placements. Evidence suggests that online learning allows for flexbility and supports learning (Liu & Wang, 2009). In addition, it provides opportunities to network and gain treatment ideas while on fieldwork. Creel (2001) reported that 89% of students involved in web-based instruction during fieldwork indicated a strong interest in participating in it again for their next Level II fieldwork.

Training Materials for Fieldwork Education

Training materials help fieldwork supervisors to guide students through the fieldwork experience. Training materials include, but are not limited to, a manual, competency checklist, site-specific objectives, and developmental timeline (Nastasi, 2014).

Manual

Fieldwork manuals provide a mechanism to store pertinent information about the fieldwork placement. The fieldwork supervisor will decide whether students should review the materials prior to the fieldwork placement or during the first week of the placement. Manuals should include a competency checklist, site-specific objectives, and a developmental timeline for the students (Nastasi, 2014).

Competency Checklist

A competency checklist lists all of the competencies that students need to complete to pass a fieldwork placement. The checklist identifies the specific requirements that the fieldwork supervisors and students should address during the fieldwork placement. The fieldwork supervisors and students should review the checklist on a weekly basis to ensure that students are making progress on the required competencies. The competency checklist should correspond to the entry-level requirements for OTs and OTAs at their site. At the end of the Level II fieldwork placement, students should achieve entry-level status.

Site-Specific Objectives

Fieldwork sites evaluate students at the middle and the end of Level II fieldwork using the *Fieldwork Performance Evaluation* (AOTA [American Occupational Therapy Association], 2002). Sites should develop site-specific objectives that align with the *Fieldwork Performance Evaluation*. Typically, sites identify specific objectives for each of the items on the evaluation. In the case where sites do not have site-specific objectives, the sites may opt to use site-specific objectives provided by the occupational therapy education program sending fieldwork students to the site. Whether the site or the educational program creates the site-specific objectives, ACOTE (2011) requires that fieldwork sites have site-specific objectives.

Developmental Timeline

Finally, fieldwork sites should provide students with a developmental timeline providing guidelines for when students should achieve milestones throughout the fieldwork experience. Timelines break down the students' responsibilities in terms of caseload and knowledge (Nastasi, 2014). Students should be carrying their supervisor's full caseload by the end of the fieldwork placement. The timeline provides students and fieldwork supervisors with a natural progression for the student's competency development while providing structure and guidance for supervision (Kleiser & Cox, 2008).

Now consider the case study. During the first week of John's fieldwork placement, he completed a formal orientation and read the site's fieldwork manual. After reading the manual, John met with his fieldwork supervisor to discuss how they would address the skills on the competency checklist, site-specific objectives, and developmental timeline. John knew that his fieldwork supervisor expected him to be responsible for half of the supervisor's caseload by the fourth week of his placement. John also knew that he would be responsible for the whole caseload by his final week of fieldwork.

Each night John wrote in his journal about his fieldwork experiences. As John approached his fourth week of fieldwork, he reread all of his entries. John realized how much he was progressing as he reread the first 4 weeks of his journal. During John's mid-term evaluation, he sat down with his supervisor and identified areas that he thought he was excelling in and areas that he felt were challenging. John and his fieldwork supervisor planned times to go over some of the areas that John felt were challenging. John's fieldwork supervisor told him that he was right on target and was carrying half of the field supervisor's caseload.

John continued to journal and work with his fieldwork supervisor on the areas that he felt were challenging at the mid-term evaluation. As John entered the last week of his fieldwork, he reread his journal entries. John realized that his meetings with his supervisor paid off. John no longer felt challenged in the areas he identified. When John and his supervisor met for his final evaluation, the fieldwork supervisor concurred. John's supervisor reported that John met all of the requirements of an entry-level OTA. John successfully completed his first Level II fieldwork placement.

TRAINING FIELDWORK SUPERVISORS

Formal training for fieldwork coordinators and fieldwork supervisors is available through the AOTA's Fieldwork Educators Certificate Workshop (AOTA, 2012). The workshop addresses administration, education, supervision, and evaluation to fieldwork coordinators and fieldwork supervisors (Nastasi, 2014). Prior to the AOTA offering this workshop, fieldwork supervisors generally receive on-the-job training to become fieldwork supervisors. Some occupational therapy education programs also provided training to the fieldwork sites where they sent their students. Training in fieldwork supervision is important because it is critical to the continued development and growth of the occupational therapy profession.

CONCLUSION

"The purpose of fieldwork education is to propel each generation of occupational therapy practitioners from the role of student to that of practitioner" (AOTA, 2009, p. 821). If occupational therapy practitioners did not supervise students, the field of occupational therapy would eventually end. Fieldwork supervisors provide the opportunity to yield the next generation of practitioners and leaders for the profession. Without future occupational therapy practitioners, societal needs would not be met (Nastasi, 2014).

SUGGESTED WEBSITES

- American Occupational Therapy Association fieldwork education resources: http://www.aota.org/en/Education-Careers/Fieldwork.aspx
- AOTA resources for new fieldwork programs: http://www.aota.org/Education-Careers/Fieldwork/NewPrograms/Steps.aspx

REVIEW QUESTIONS

1. The _____ is responsible for placing students on Level I and Level II fieldwork placements.

    a. Fieldwork coordinator

    b. Fieldwork educator

    c. Fieldwork supervisor

    d. Fieldwork site

2. The _____ is responsible for supervising students on Level I and Level II fieldwork placements.

    a. Fieldwork coordinator

    b. Fieldwork educator

    c. Fieldwork supervisor

    d. Fieldwork site

3. The_____ may supervise occupational therapy students on Level II fieldwork.

    a. OT

    b. OTA

    c. Occupational therapy aide

    d. Occupational therapy practitioners

4. The _____ may supervise OTA students on Level II fieldwork.

    a. OT

    b. OTA

    c. Occupational therapy aide

    d. Occupational therapy practitioners

5. The _____ may supervise occupational therapy students on Level I fieldwork.

    a. OT

    b. OTA

    c. Occupational therapy aide

    d. Occupational therapy practitioners

6. The _____ may supervise OTA students on Level I fieldwork.

    a. OT

    b. OTA

    c. Occupational therapy aide

    d. Occupational therapy practitioners

7. How many years of practice do occupational therapy practitioners need to supervise students on fieldwork?

    a. Less than 1 year of practice

    b. 1 year of practice

    c. 2 years of practice

    d. 3 years of practice

8. The goal of Level I fieldwork education is to:

    a. Provide hands-on experience

    b. Provide observational experience

    c. Create entry-level practitioners

    d. Replace lab activities

9. The goal of Level II fieldwork is to:

    a. Provide hands-on experience

    b. Provide observational experience

    c. Create entry-level practitioners

    d. Replace lab activities

10. True or false: Students must complete at least one Level I or Level II fieldwork placement in a setting that addresses psychosocial needs of the client.

    a. True

    b. False

REFERENCES

Accreditation Council for Occupational Therapy Education. (2011). 2011 *Accreditation Council for Occupational Therapy Education (ACOTE*®*) Standards and Interpretive Guide*. Bethesda, MD: ACOTE.

American Occupational Therapy Association. (2002). *Fieldwork performance evaluation for occupational therapy students*. Bethesda, MD.

American Occupational Therapy Association. (2009). Occupational therapy fieldwork education: Value and purpose. *American Journal of Occupational Therapy, 63*, 821-822.

American Occupational Therapy Association. (2012). *Fieldwork educators certificate workshop*. Retrieved from http://www.aota.org/Educate/EdRes/Fieldwork/Workshop.aspx

Buchanan, H., van Niekerk, L., & Moore, R. (2001). Assessing fieldwork journals: Developmental portfolios. *British Journal of Occupational Therapy, 64*, 398-402.

Bonello, M. (2001). Fieldwork within the context of higher education: A literature review. *British Journal of Occupational Therapy, 64*, 93-99.

Creel, T. (2001). Chat rooms and level II fieldwork. *Occupational Therapy in Health Care, 14*, 55-59.

Duke, L. (2004). Piecing together the jigsaw: How do practice educators define occupational therapy student competence? *British Journal of Occupational Therapy, 67*, 201-209.

Gutman, S. A., McCreedy, P., & Heisler, P. (1998). Student level II fieldwork: Strategies for intervention. *American Journal of Occupational Therapy, 52*, 143-149.

Holloway, E. L., & Neufeldt, S. A. (1995). Supervision: Its contributions to treatment efficacy. *Journal of Consulting and Clinical Psychology, 63*, 207-213.

Kirke, P., Layton, N., & Sims, J. (2007). Informing fieldwork design: Key elements to quality in fieldwork education for undergraduate occupational therapy students. *Australian Occupational Therapy Journal, 54*, S13-S22.

Kleiser, H., & Cox, D. L. (2008). The integration of clinical and managerial supervision: A critical literature review. *British Journal of Occupational Therapy, 71*, 2-9.

Liu, Y., & Wang, H. (2009). A comparative study on e-learning technologies and products: From the east to the west. *Systems Research and Behavioral Science, 26*, 191-209.

Maizel, M., Yerkes, E., Macejko, A., Hagerty, J., Chaviano, A. H., Cheng, E. Y., . . . Kaplan, W. E. (2008). A new computer enhanced visual learning method to train urology residents in pediatric orchiopexy: A prototype for accreditation council for graduate medical education. *Journal of Urology, 180,* 1814-1818.

Nastasi, J. (2012). Specialty level II fieldwork in low vision rehabilitation. *OT Practice, 17*(11), 13-16.

Nastasi, J. (2014). Fieldwork education. In K. Jacobs, N. MacRae, & K. Sladyk (Eds.), *Occupational therapy essentials for clinical practice* (2nd ed., pp. 559-565). Thorofare, NJ: SLACK Incorporated.

NBCOT [National Board for Certification in Occupational Therapy]. (2009). *Eligibility requirements.* Retrieved from http://nbcot.org/index.php?option=com_content&view=article&id=247&Itemid=154

Nolinske, T. (1995). Multiple mentoring relationships facilitate learning during fieldwork. *American Journal of Occupational Therapy, 49,* 39-43.

Robertson, L. J., & Griffiths, S. (2009). Graduate's reflections on their preparation for practice. *British Journal of Occupational Therapy, 72,* 125-132.

Thomas, Y., Dickson, D., Broadbridge, J., Hopper, L., Hawkins, R., Edwards, A., & McBryde, C. (2007). Benefits and challenges of supervising occupational therapy fieldwork students: Supervisor's perspectives. *Australian Occupational Therapy Journal, 54,* S2-S12.

9

Communication Skills
Health Literacy

Nancy W. Doyle, OTD, OTR/L

ACOTE Standard explored in this chapter:

- B.5.18. Demonstrate an understanding of health literacy and the ability to educate and train the client, caregiver, family, and significant others to facilitate skills in areas of occupation as well as prevention, health maintenance, health promotion, and safety.

KEY VOCABULARY

Communication skills: Skills used to communicate so that we understand and are understood by our clients.

Health literacy: The ability to find, understand, and use information to make health-related decisions.

Learner characteristics: Features of a learner that may influence his or her learning experience and retention of information.

Health literacy environment: Characteristics of an environment that support or hinder health literacy.

eHealth literacy: Electronic health literacy, or the ability to find, understand, and use information obtained from electronic resources (e.g., Internet search) to make health-related decisions.

Jacobs K, ed.
Management and Administration for the OTA:
Leadership and Application Skills (pp 117-129).
© 2016 Taylor & Francis Group.

CASE STUDY

You are working with Nadia, a kindergartener with poor core and hand strength who is having particular difficulty with fine motor skills and pre-writing readiness. Her occupational therapy evaluation did not indicate any significant difficulties with sensory processing, self-regulation, or behavior. Her treatment plan includes immediate adaptations to support her pre-writing readiness and ability to sit up in class and occupation-based interventions to increase her abdominal, back, upper extremity, hand, and finger strength.

Nadia is an early reader, with the ability to read simple words and numbers 1 to 10. Her grandmother is the caregiver who has the most regular contact with you. You notice that her grandmother often complains of forgetting her glasses, wears a hearing aid, and says that she prefers to watch television rather than read—whether with Nadia or in her own leisure time. She says that, in her home country, she had never heard of occupational therapy. She also says that this is her first experience with occupational therapy and does not quite understand what abdominal strength is or how occupational therapy will help Nadia in kindergarten. When you provide home programs for Nadia, you realize that she usually returns the following week having practiced only the first exercise on the list.

Good communication is integral to our therapeutic use of self as occupational therapy assistants (OTAs). We use skills like active listening, acceptance, and confidentiality to communicate effectively with our clients (Moss, 2012). Such communication skills help us develop and sustain our therapeutic relationships, express empathy, and collaborate effectively with our clients (American Occupational Therapy Association [AOTA], 2014). Communication is ongoing, dynamic, and dependent on all parties involved in the conversation. We are responsible to "facilitate meaningful communication and comprehension" (AOTA, 2010, p. 6; 2014), in accordance with our professional code of ethics. In other words, we must communicate clearly so that we understand and are understood by our clients.

We need to ensure that our clients understand the health information we are sharing with them. How we communicate this information affects whether and how our clients "achieve health, well-being, and participation in life through engagement in occupation" (AOTA, 2014, p. S4)—the essence of occupational therapy practice. Much of the "how" of our communication depends on the health literacy of our clients and of ourselves as health practitioners (United States Department of Health and Human Services [USDHHS], 2010). In this chapter, we will define health literacy and discuss how occupational therapy practitioners use this concept to better understand the client, the client's health environment, and the client's occupations and health activities.

HEALTH LITERACY: CLIENT PERSPECTIVE

Health literacy is the "degree to which individuals can obtain, process, and understand the basic health information and services they need to make appropriate health decisions" (Institute of Medicine [IOM], 2004, p. 1). A 2004 report by the Institute of Medicine indicates that 90 million Americans, or nearly half of the adult population of the United States, have low health literacy (IOM, 2004). In fact, limited health literacy may affect up to 90% of English-speaking adults in the United States (USDHHS, 2010). As the use of computer and Internet health-related tools increases, not just health literacy but also eHealth literacy, or electronic health literacy, is important (Brown & Dickson, 2010). Research indicates that low health literacy may affect the health of individuals, as well as the ability of the health care system to provide quality care (IOM, 2004). For individual clients, low health literacy may negatively affect the use of preventative services and the self-management of chronic disease (Bendycki, 2008). Low health literacy may even be associated with increased mortality after other sociodemographic and health factors have been accounted for (Bendycki, 2008). It is part of our professional responsibility to address this public health issue both at an individual treatment level and at a systematic health services level (Egbert & Nanna, 2009; USDHHS, 2010).

Health literacy is not just about the ability to read and understand written health-related information. Health literacy also includes skills in writing, numeracy, listening, speaking, and conceptual knowledge (IOM, 2004). For example, when an individual receives a prescription for medicine, she must understand that she should take the prescription to the pharmacy to fill it (writing and conceptual knowledge). She needs to read the written and/or verbal instructions provided by the doctor and pharmacist about taking the medication (writing, listening). She must understand when and how many pills to take (numeracy) and ask questions about the medication, dosage, and duration of the prescription (speaking). In addition, it is important that the client understand the reason for and importance of the medicine (conceptual knowledge). Finally, the client must go one step further and ultimately use the health materials and information as intended (Egbert & Nanna, 2009).

Now consider our case study. In it, you have the literacy of two people to consider. Nadia is a young child with emerging skills in reading and numeracy. Her grandmother wears a hearing aid and so may have a hearing impairment. She also expresses limited conceptual knowledge of occupational therapy. Finally, her comments about forgetting her glasses, preferring television, and working on only the first of any home program exercises indicates that writing may be a difficult mode of acquiring health information to assist her granddaughter.

HEALTH LITERACY: PRACTITIONER PERSPECTIVE

There is an additional component of health literacy to consider, and this is on the side of the health professional. Health literacy "depends upon the skills, preferences, and expectations of health information and care providers" (IOM, 2004, p. 1). In our first example, what are the expectations of the doctor prescribing the medication and the pharmacist filling the prescription?

As an OTA or OTA student, you must "demonstrate an understanding of health literacy and the ability to educate and train the client, caregiver, and family and significant others to facilitate skills in areas of occupation as well as prevention, health maintenance, health promotion, and safety" (Accreditation Council for Occupational Therapy Education [ACOTE], 2013, p. 26). In our case study with Nadia, what are your health literacy expectations, skills, and preferences as an occupational therapy practitioner? That is, what are your preferences for sharing information about health and occupational therapy? What are your expectations of what Nadia and her grandmother should or can be doing at home to support her work in occupational therapy sessions? Most critically, how can you align your expectations, skills, and preferences with the health literacy and learning needs of Nadia and her grandmother?

We will continue to explore these concepts as we take a further look at health literacy and the learning process of our clients.

UNDERSTANDING OUR CLIENTS

Our work affords many active teaching and learning opportunities regarding occupation, health, and participation (AOTA, 2007). For example, we may teach a client one-handed adaptations for cooking, a group of home health aides about proper lifting techniques, and populations with severe mental illness about the physical and mental benefits of occupational engagement. In each scenario and at each client level, we must strive to provide the most effective, efficient, and health-literate teaching-learning process for our clients. Just as in all areas of occupational therapy practice, our challenge is to provide not only the best clinical intervention, but also the best education possible that is guided by theory, based in evidence, and infused with our clinical reasoning (AOTA, 2010, 2014).

Each client, whether as a population, group, or individual, has a unique capacity to communicate and comprehend health information. We can look at several learner characteristics to better understand each client's capacity for health literacy. These characteristics can be grouped together in what we might call a learner profile. Two main questions guide the development of these profiles: (1) what are the clients' learning needs? and (2) what are the learning characteristics of our clients? First, we must determine with clients and their significant others what they need to know. Then, we work to understand characteristics of these learners so we can develop the most successful learning experience possible. These profiles consider the specific abilities, readiness, and motivation of the learners. They also include evaluation of the developmental and literacy levels of the learners.

Learner Needs

To create successful learning experiences for our clients, we must first work with them to determine their learning needs. These are the information, processes, adaptations, habits, and routines the client needs to achieve or enhance his or her occupational goals. For example, if a client is recovering from a rotator-cuff tear and has a goal to return to cooking daily meals for his family, he may have a need to learn one-handed adaptations in the kitchen and recipe shortcuts. If a business is working with an occupational therapy practitioner to reduce work-related injuries, learning needs may include ergonomic information and education about the importance of new work habits such as regular rest and stretch breaks. If an OTA is contributing to public health efforts to combat childhood obesity, he or she may provide education about occupational balance, as well as the importance of providing not only discussion of, but also actual opportunities within, a program for building new routines that incorporate physical activity, healthy cooking and eating, and rest and leisure occupations. For our case study, what are Nadia's learning needs and what are those of her grandmother? Nadia and her grandmother both need information about adaptations and building Nadia's strength, but her grandmother may also need additional education about occupational therapy and how it can help Nadia succeed in her kindergarten classroom. Once learning needs such as these have been determined, other learner characteristics can be examined to plan the best client education possible.

Learner Abilities

As we work with clients, we are looking for their abilities, strengths, and challenges. Perhaps the client has strong visual skills but difficulty with multi-step directions. Or the client self-regulates attention levels well but has difficulty hearing. As you take note of client factors, performance skills, and performance patterns that affect a client's occupational performance, you will see that many of the same abilities, strengths, and challenges will also impact the client's health literacy and ability to learn.

In addition to learning abilities that would be evaluated during the occupational therapy process (AOTA, 2014), additional considerations may include cognitive and learning styles. While both style types will benefit from continued basic and applied research to better understand the constructs and their application in educational settings (Coffield, Moseley, Hall, & Ecclestone, 2004; Kozhevnikov, 2007; Pashler, McDaniel, Rohrer, & Bjork, 2009; Peterson, Rayner, & Armstrong, 2009), a basic understanding of their concepts allows occupational therapy professionals to further tailor learning experiences to the strengths and abilities of their clients.

Cognitive styles are generally defined as relatively stable ways of processing information from an individual's environment (Kozhevnikov, 2007). They include whether an individual tends to focus holistically or analytically on new information. For example, does a client prefer to discuss the whole occupational therapy process—from evaluation to intervention to outcomes—initially or would the client prefer to focus on just one aspect at a time? Another cognitive style, termed *field (in)dependence*, looks at whether a person relies heavily on the environment to interpret information. Someone who relies heavily on environmental cues may benefit from working in a group setting where social cues may enhance the intervention process.

Learning styles and preferences are factors that affect learning behavior specifically. The Experiential Learning Theory (Kolb & Kolb, 2005) describes learning as a process where a skill is grasped through concrete experience or abstract conceptualization and then transformed into new knowledge for an individual through reflective observation or active experimentation. In other words, a client may prefer to consider home modifications to prevent falls by actively practicing these strategies in the clinic or by more abstractly talking through them with an occupational therapy practitioner. Then, the client may prefer to take some time to reflect on these strategies before implementing them, or may prefer to experiment with these strategies at home between occupational therapy sessions.

Clients may have preferences for the perceptual mode in which they learn. Some clients may prefer to learn visually with pictures and diagrams, aurally through audio recordings or discussions, visually through reading written text, or kinesthetically through active manipulation of learning materials (Fleming & Bonwell, 2006). For example, clients may prefer to complete a home program with a video, written guide, or audio guide, depending on their learning preferences. For Nadia and her grandmother, would a handout with pictures of home program exercises be useful? Would a video of home programming be helpful, especially since Nadia's grandmother has stated that this is her preferred method of entertainment?

Learner Readiness

After understanding the learning needs and abilities of clients, it is important to assess their readiness. The client must see a need to learn what is being taught and be ready to engage in the learning process. Readiness to learn will be affected by a variety of factors both internal and external to the client. Because learning depends on readiness levels in different parts of the brain (National Research Council, 2000), internally the individual's systems, especially sensory systems, need to be functioning at an appropriate level so that information can be both received and processed (Ayres, 1973). Cognitive, emotional, and psychological readiness are also aspects of learner readiness. For example, clients who are currently stressed by an acute health problem may find their readiness to learn and their ability to retain information affected (Gustafsson, Hodge, Robinson, McKenna, & Bower, 2010). Externally, it is important to determine whether the context and conditions for working with a client are also ready for the teaching-learning process. If the environment is too noisy or the number of sessions is limited, it is important to consider what learning can be completed in these scenarios with a client who is ready to engage in the teaching-learning process.

For Nadia, you will want to determine whether she is ready to accept adaptations to compensate for her strength deficits in the short term. You will also want to see if she is ready to engage in strength-building exercises and occupations to develop her own strength for classroom and school-related activities. For Nadia's grandmother, you will want to try to understand whether she is ready to learn about occupational therapy and its relevance to school performance, as well as Nadia's specific health needs.

Learner Motivation

Motivation, as well as readiness, facilitates the teaching-learning process. When a client is both able to grasp new learning and motivated to do so, learning will be more successful. Clients may be motivated extrinsically by rewards or consequences; motivation may be intrinsic such that clients engage in learning for their own satisfaction or self-improvement. Generally, intrinsic motivation is most potent (Radel, Sarrazin, Legrain, & Wild, 2010). If the new learning is personally relevant, functional, or utilitarian or contributes to helping others, it is often more meaningful to the learner. In addition, materials that are neither too hard nor too easy, but instead are at the "just-right challenge" for a client, will avoid frustration or boredom and promote motivation. Motivation can also be contagious; learners often become motivated to learn if they sense genuine excitement and investment in the teaching-learning process by instructors or their peers (Radel et al., 2010). This speaks to the potential power of occupational therapy professionals and peers to motivate learners in a wide variety of contexts, including group treatment and community settings. For Nadia, consider whether she will be motivated by her own successes, will need some external rewards from you as the occupational therapy professional, or would benefit from a group setting where she can engage with and be motivated by peers, as well as group leaders.

Developmental Stages of Learning

Identifying the developmental level at which a client functions will help the occupational therapy practitioner tailor the teaching-learning process appropriately. Development from infancy through old age must be considered (Bastable & Dart, 2011), including typical development, delays in development, and possible regression in the case of an injury or illness, such as brain injury or dementia. Psychosocial and cognitive development are commonly considered. In order, Ericson's stages of psychosocial development focus on the development of trust, autonomy, initiative, industry, identity, intimacy, generativity, and ego integrity (Bastable & Dart, 2011). Piaget's stages of cognitive development look at learning from sensorimotor, preoperational, concrete operations, and formal operations perspectives (Piaget, 1954). When working with an infant, the focus may be on developing trust in new movement patterns through exploring toys with the therapist and caretakers; when working with an adult, a more abstract discussion of roles and routines may help a client consider his or her contributions, successes, and areas for modification in occupational plans for the future. Nadia and her grandmother are at opposite ends of the developmental spectrum in terms of age and so you will want to consider different levels of psychosocial and cognitive development when planning your communication and education for each of them.

Literacy Level

Assessing the learning needs of a client includes determining the client's literacy level. This includes gathering information about the client's primary language for communication and his or her general ability to comprehend spoken and written language. Smith and Gutman (2011) report that the average American reads at a sixth-grade level, much lower than the tenth-grade level in which most information is communicated. This indicates a huge gap in what we say or write and what our clients may understand. We have a responsibility to be sure that what we communicate is at the appropriate literacy level so that our clients are able to fully grasp the information we provide to them.

Health Literacy

When it comes to health literacy specifically, we should remember that approximately half of all Americans have low health literacy. That is, they have "difficulty understanding and acting on health information" (Smith & Gutman, 2011, p. 367). In fact, some reports indicate that only 12%

of Americans have adequate health literacy to access, understand, and utilize health information (Egbert & Nanna, 2009). We want to assess health literacy confidentially and informally. Formal testing of literacy skills may upset or isolate some clients. Instead, a question such as, "How confident are you filling out medical forms by yourself?" (Cornett, 2009, p. 5) may be sufficient for determining that a client could benefit from assistance with health information. Additional behavioral cues (Cornett, 2009) may include avoiding reading pamphlets or filling out forms while in occupational therapy sessions, the client stating that she has forgotten her glasses, that her eyes are tired, or that she will do this at home. Clients with low literacy may not complete intake forms, or may do so incorrectly. When provided written information, their eyes may wander over but not focus on reading material. Clients with low literacy may miss appointments and may be anxious, confused, or indifferent with written and health information. As you consider our case study, are you noticing any of these behavioral cues by Nadia or her grandmother? By attending to such potential indicators of low literacy, we can choose words and educational materials most appropriate to the literacy needs of our clients in our teaching-learning process.

THE CLIENT'S HEALTH ENVIRONMENT

After looking at clients' specific learning characteristics and health literacy status, it is useful to look more broadly at the health environment around them. We want to consider three main contextual perspectives: that of the client, that of the practitioner, and that of the setting where client and practitioner interact.

First, we want to understand our clients' context and culture. This will help to situate their learning needs and appropriately design culturally sensitive teaching approaches. It is important to examine the cultural, personal, temporal, virtual, physical, and social contexts (AOTA, 2014) of clients and consider their relation to client education. Understanding whether a company works on a traditional 8-hour day or uses a different temporal rhythm for workers can impact how and when an occupational therapy practitioner provides educational sessions for administration and staff. For example, when working with refugee women from another country, it is important to understand their cultural roles, expectations, and aspirations. Whether their cultural context is based on a matriarchy or patriarchy can, for example, affect how new information is presented and whether it is presented just to the women or also to men. When working to promote healthy occupational participation for at-risk youth, it is important to note whether the physical environment includes, for example, safe playgrounds, community centers, or libraries that could promote healthy occupational choices.

Next, it is important that we consider our own context and culture and how these characteristics impact the way we communicate about health with our clients. What are our assumptions about health and health promotion? How do we view occupation and occupational engagement as influencing health and quality of life? Our answers to these important questions may be very different than those of our clients. An awareness of our own background and assumptions about health will help us determine any differences from our clients in approaches, attitudes, health literacy, and desired health and occupational outcomes.

Finally, it is important to be attuned to the context in which we are interacting with the client. Earlier, we explored how the learning environment may affect learner readiness. As occupational therapy practitioners, we are used to analyzing how a variety of contextual and environmental characteristics are affecting the learning and occupational engagement of our clients. For example, a noisy environment may stimulate a learning experience for some individuals and impede learning for others, who perform better in a quiet setting.

In addition to these characteristics, it is important to consider the health literacy characteristics of the learning environment. For example, are a variety of client education materials available? Are materials presented at different literacy levels? Are they available in print, audio, and video formats? In addition, do health professionals interact with clients in a health-literate manner? Are explanations communicated in everyday language for all clients or is professional jargon commonplace? Are health professionals able to tailor their communication based on different health literacy needs and developmental stages of clients?

Creating a Health-Literate Environment

Research literature provides several examples of how client education can be tailored to best fit the health literacy needs of different individuals and populations. That is, communicating with clients in an evidence-based, health-literate manner. Some recent literature points to the importance of providing information about a client's health conditions and how to manage them as part of client education (Radomski, Davidson, Voydetich, & Erickson, 2009). For example, Radomski and colleagues (2009) report that clients with mild traumatic brain injury who received information about their health condition, as well as therapeutic interventions during occupational therapy sessions, reported fewer symptoms and shorter symptom duration.

The occupational therapy literature in areas such as stroke rehabilitation (Gustafsson et al., 2010), adult physical disabilities (Sharry, McKenna, & Tooth, 2002), and mild traumatic brain injury (Radomski et al., 2009) emphasizes the importance of providing multisensory and repetitious learning opportunities for clients. That is, clients can benefit from information being presented verbally as well as in written formats (Radomski et al., 2009; Sharry et al., 2002) and from demonstration of and active practice or engagement with new learning (Gustafsson et al., 2010). Repetition of the new information may be useful for some learners. Some clients may benefit from teaching opportunities that are provided across occupational therapy sessions, particularly if their cognitive or other learning capacities increase over time or their learning needs change as they progress through various stages of therapy (Gustafsson et al., 2010).

When considering a client at the group or population level, it seems particularly important to provide learning opportunities that target a variety of learning preferences. This will provide a more inclusive learning experience for clients with different health literacy levels and learning and cognitive styles within the targeted group or population.

Finally, some authors have argued that the best way to promote health literacy for all clients is to be sure all of our communication, services, and materials are universally accessible to everyone (Egbert & Nanna, 2009; Levasseur & Carrier, 2012; USDHHS, 2010). That is, our client communication should be culturally appropriate, use plain language, and be delivered using appropriate media (Egbert & Nanna, 2009). We can use stories as a health literacy tool to explain health information or evidence-based practice information in an understandable and engaging manner (Arbesman & Lieberman, 2014). We can check that we are communicating with clients at a level appropriate to their health literacy capabilities by using different strategies, such as "Ask Me 3" and "Teach Back" (Bendycki, 2008). In "Ask Me 3," we want clients to be able to answer these three questions: (1) what is my main problem? (2) what do I need to do? and (3) why is it important for me to do this? (Bendycki, 2008). In the "Teach Back" method, we ask clients (1) what they would tell family or friends about what was discussed in this session, (2) what they felt was most important in the discussion, and (3) what they heard you as an occupational therapy practitioner say—to help you know whether you gave clients the information they wanted and needed in this session (Bendycki, 2008). For Nadia and her grandmother, it will be important to ask each of them what they learned that day. You may also ask them to describe, for example, what they would tell Nadia's parents or other caregivers about her occupational therapy session and that week's home program.

As part of our client-centered care, it is critical that we check on the clarity and effectiveness of our communication with the clients themselves. It is also important that we make this an interdisciplinary effort whenever we collaborate with other professionals to serve the health and occupational needs of our clients (Levasseur & Carrier, 2012). Addressing their health literacy needs and capabilities contributes to our provision of effective, accessible health information for our clients.

By addressing health literacy concerns and levels universally as a standard of our occupational therapy practice, we are also promoting health literacy at a broader and more systematic level (Levasseur & Carrier, 2012).

CLIENT OCCUPATIONS AND HEALTH ACTIVITIES

After analyzing the clients' health literacy level and environment, we shift our focus to how our interactions with them can promote their occupational engagement and participation in health activities and their health literacy capabilities. We need to be sure that our services include advancing their health literacy, if necessary. For example, if a client with diabetes is unable to read and follow multi-step directions to test insulin levels and take medication appropriately, we have a role in improving their ability to carry out these health-promoting activities. Just as we complete activity analyses to determine client needs in their daily occupations, we can "deconstruct health activities" (Smith & Gutman, 2011, p. 368) and how they interact with clients' unique environments. We can then work with clients to educate them in the difficult areas of their health activities, thereby increasing intervention effectiveness (Smith & Gutman, 2011) and supporting clients' abilities to make appropriate and optimal health choices (Pizur-Barnekow & Darragh, 2011).

Learning Objectives

For some clients, improving aspects of their health literacy may be done concretely by setting health literacy goals and objectives as part of their overall occupational therapy intervention plan. As with other goals and objectives, these would be developed collaboratively between the occupational therapist and client, with input from OTAs and the client's significant others, as appropriate.

When setting these goals and objectives, it is important to consider not only the content of what the client desires to learn, but also the timing and sequence of the teaching-learning process. For example, the learning objectives may describe when new health information will first be presented and how often it will be reinforced in the provision of therapy services (Gustafsson et al., 2010). Learning objectives should include (1) where the learning will take place, (2) the duration of the teaching-learning process, (3) what the learner will demonstrate at the end of the teaching-learning process, and (4) how well the learner will perform at the end of the teaching-learning process.

Additional considerations for learning objectives might include whether the new knowledge or skill will be transferred to new situations or occupations. The amount of time and the pace of learning should be considered in relation to the complexity or volume of material and the client's learning characteristics. The amount of practice needed to master new aspects of occupational performance should also be considered when writing learning objectives and carrying out the teaching-learning process.

MEETING HEALTH LITERACY NEEDS

As in all areas of practice, it is important to determine whether health literacy goals and objectives have been met. OTAs work with clients and supervising OTs to assess progress with objectives. Questions that need to be addressed are (1) Were health literacy objectives met? (2) How has addressing health literacy needs affected occupational performance and health? and (3) Is more client education needed to reach a level of health literacy where clients can utilize health information appropriately? Gaining the client's perception of health literacy needs and capabilities provides valuable information for future sessions and encourages self-reflection by the client. Pre- and post-test assessments may provide valuable information about the teaching-learning process. For example, the Canadian Occupational Performance Measure (Law et al., 1998) can reflect elements of the new learning as clients report on whether their satisfaction and performance of prioritized areas of health literacy and occupational performance have improved. When working with families or significant others, good communication skills, time to absorb the material presented, and time for questions become critical for carryover at home. Taking such time for clear communication can facilitate clients' understanding of the critical concepts presented and improve the likelihood of appropriate application. The success of occupational therapy and health literacy education hinges on a meaningful understanding of what is being taught and the ability to transfer that knowledge to situations when it is needed.

CONCLUSION

This chapter has presented an overview of some of the important issues involved in communication skills and health literacy. These include understanding clients' health literacy levels, needs, and capabilities. It explored the health literacy characteristics of client and practitioner environments. Finally, it analyzed clients' health occupations and activities, including developing and meeting health literacy learning objectives. Occupational therapy practitioners need to be aware of these issues, understand them, and incorporate them into their clinical and educational interventions for clients, families, students, colleagues, and the general public. Doing this allows for the development of optimal health literacy environments and interventions, ones that foster successful access to, understanding of, evaluation of, and communication of health information (Levasseur & Carrier, 2012) for enhanced health and well-being of our clients and the public health of our larger society.

SUGGESTED WEBSITES

- The National Institute of Health's Clear Communication Initiative: http://www.nih.gov/clearcommunication/healthliteracy.htm
- USDHHS Health Resources and Services Administration: http://www.hrsa.gov/publichealth/healthliteracy/index.html
- Centers for Disease Control and Prevention Health Literacy: http://www.cdc.gov/healthliteracy/
- Health Literacy Consulting: www.healthliteracy.com
- National Assessment of Adult Literacy: http://nces.ed.gov/naal

REVIEW QUESTIONS

1. Communication skills include:
    a. Confidentiality
    b. Active listening
    c. Acceptance
    d. All of the above

2. Communication is dependent on:
   a. The occupational therapy practitioner
   b. The client and significant others
   c. All parties involved in the conversation
   d. Face-to-face interaction

3. Health literacy includes:
   a. Obtaining health information
   b. Processing health information
   c. Understanding health information
   d. All of the above in order to make health decisions

4. Limited health literacy affects:
   a. 25% of English-speaking adults in the United States
   b. 50% of English-speaking adults in the United States
   c. 75% of English-speaking adults in the United States
   d. 90% of English-speaking adults in the United States

5. Health literacy includes:
   a. Writing
   b. Writing and numeracy
   c. Writing, numeracy, and speaking
   d. Writing, numeracy, listening, speaking, conceptual knowledge, and using health information as it was intended

6. Which of the following behavioral cues may indicate low health literacy?
   a. Always scheduling appointments on Mondays
   b. Frequently missing appointments
   c. Filling out forms in all-capital letters
   d. Using glasses to read or fill out forms

7. A client's health environment includes:
   a. The client's context and culture
   b. The practitioner's context and culture
   c. The setting where client and practitioner interact
   d. All of the above

8. We can address health literacy at a public health or systemic level by:
   a. Ensuring that all communication at our worksite is done in simple or plain language
   b. Making communication culturally relevant
   c. Using varied media for communication and tailoring this to clients' specific needs or desires
   d. All of the above

9. We can promote clients' health literacy by:

    a. Making sure they have the health literacy to engage in health activities and occupations

    b. Sharing appropriate health-related websites

    c. Tailoring communication or making it universally accessible

    d. Both a and c

10. Health literacy is:

    a. A public health issue

    b. Important for all professionals who work with clients on health-related issues

    c. Important for occupational therapy practitioners to be aware of and address with clients

    d. All of the above

REFERENCES

Accreditation Council for Occupational Therapy Education. (2013). 2011 Accreditation Council for Occupational Therapy Education (ACOTE®) Standards and Interpretive Guide (effective July 31, 2013) December 2014 Interpretive Guide Version. Retrieved from: http://www.aota.org/-/media/Corporate/Files/EducationCareers/Accredit/Standards/2011-Standards-and-Interpretive-Guide.pdf

American Occupational Therapy Association. (2007). Philosophy of occupational therapy education. *American Journal of Occupational Therapy, 61,* 678.

American Occupational Therapy Association. (2010). Occupational therapy code of ethics and ethics standards. *American Journal of Occupational Therapy, 64,* S14-S24.

American Occupational Therapy Association. (2014). Occupational therapy practice framework: Domain and process (3rd ed.). *American Journal of Occupational Therapy, 68*(Suppl. 1), S1-S48. http://dx.doi.org/10.5014/ajot.2014.682006.

Arbesman, M., & Lieberman, D. (2014). Using stories to communicate evidence. *OT Practice, 19*(9), 7, 20.

Ayres, A. J. (1973). *Sensory integration and learning disorders.* Los Angeles, CA: Western Psychological Services.

Bastable, S. B., & Dart, M. A. (2011). Developmental stages of the learner. In S. B. Bastable., P. Gramet, K. Jacobs, & D. L. Sopczyk (Eds.), *Health professional as educator: Principles of teaching and learning* (pp. 151-197). Sudbury, MA: Jones & Bartlett Learning.

Bendycki, N. A. (2008). Health literacy. *Marketing Health Services,* 2008 (Fall), 32-37.

Brown, C. A., & Dickson, R. D. (2010). Healthcare students' e-literacy skills. Journal of Allied Health, 39(3), 179-184.

Coffield, F., Moseley, D., Hall, E., & Ecclestone, K. (2004). *Learning styles and pedagogy in post-16 learning: A systematic and critical review.* London: Learning and Skills Research Centre.

Cornett, S. (2009). Assessing and addressing health literacy. *OJIN: Online Journal of Issues in Nursing, 14,* manuscript 2.

Egbert, N., & Nanna, K. M. (2009). Health literacy: Challenges and strategies. *OJIN: Online Journal of Issues in Nursing, 14*(3), 5.

Fleming, N. D., & Bonwell, C. C. (2006). *VARK questionnaire, version 7.0.* Retrieved from http://www.vark-learn.com/english/page.asp?p=questionnaire

Gustafsson, L., Hodge, A., Robinson, M., McKenna, K., & Bower, K. (2010). Information provision to clients with stroke and their carers: Self-reported practices of occupational therapists. *Australian Occupational Therapy Journal, 57,* 190-196.

Institute of Medicine. (2004). *Health literacy: A prescription to end confusion.* Washington, DC: National Academies Press.

Kolb, A. Y., & Kolb, D. A. (2005). *The Kolb Learning Style Inventory: Version 3.1 2005 technical specifications.* Boston: Hay Resources Direct.

Kozhevnikov, M. (2007). Cognitive styles in the context of modern psychology: Toward an integrated framework of cognitive style. *Psychological Bulletin, 133,* 464-481.

Law, M., Baptiste, S., Carswell, A., McColl, M. A., Polatajko, H., & Pollock, N. (1998). *Canadian occupational performance measure* (3rd ed.). Thorofare, NJ: SLACK Incorporated.

Levasseur, M., & Carrier, A. (2012). *Integrating health literacy into occupational therapy: Findings from a scoping review.* Scandinavian Journal of Occupational Therapy, 19, 305-314. doi:10.3109/11038128.2011.588724.

Moss, B. (2012). *Communication skills in health and social care* (2nd ed.). London: SAGE Publications Ltd.

National Research Council. (2000). *How people learn: Brain mind, experience and school, expanded edition.* Washington, DC: National Academy Press.

Pashler, H., McDaniel, M., Rohrer, D., & Bjork, R. (2009). Learning styles: Concepts and evidence. *Psychological Science in the Public Interest, 9,* 105-119.

Peterson, E. R., Rayner, S. G., & Armstrong, S. J. (2009). Researching the psychology of cognitive style and learning style: Is there really a future? *Learning and Individual Differences, 19,* 518-523.

Piaget, J. (1954). *The construction of reality in the child.* New York: Norton.

Pizur-Barnekow, K., & Darragh, A. (2011). *AOTA's societal statement on health literacy.* Retrieved from http://www. aota.org/Practitioners/Official/SocietalStmts/Health-Literacy.aspx?FT=.pdf

Radel, R., Sarrazin, P., Legrain, P., & Wild, T. C. (2010). Social contagion of motivation between teacher and student: Analyzing underlying processes. *Journal of Educational Psychology, 102,* 577-587.

Radomski, M. V., Davidson, L., Voydetich, D., & Erickson, M. W. (2009). Occupational therapy for service members with mild traumatic brain injury. *American Journal of Occupational Therapy, 64,* 646-655.

Sharry, R., McKenna, K., & Tooth, L. (2002). Brief report: Occupational therapists' use and perceptions of written client education materials. *American Journal of Occupational Therapy, 56,* 573-576.

Smith, D. L., & Gutman, S. A. (2011). Health literacy in occupational therapy practice and research. *American Journal of Occupational Therapy, 65,* 367-369.

United States Department of Health and Human Services. (2010). *National action plan to improve health literacy.* Washington, DC: Author.

10

Ethics

Kimberly Erler, MS, OTR/L

ACOTE Standard explored in this chapter:

- B.9.1. Demonstrate knowledge and understanding of the American Occupational Therapy Association (AOTA) *Occupational Therapy Code of Ethics and Ethics Standards* and the AOTA *Standards of Practice* and use them as a guide for ethical decision-making in professional interactions, client interventions, and employment settings.

KEY VOCABULARY

Ethical principles: A set of norms that are derived from common morality.

Professional integrity: The practice of consistently acting in an honest manner while upholding moral standards of the profession.

Moral distress: The experience of knowing the ethically appropriate action but feeling powerless or constrained to implement it by external factors.

Moral courage: The willingness to uphold moral and ethical values despite the risk of criticism or negative feedback.

Preventative ethics: A strategy of implementing system-based changes to thwart common ethical issues from arising.

Jacobs K, ed.
*Management and Administration for the OTA:
Leadership and Application Skills* (pp 131-142).
© 2016 Taylor & Francis Group.

CASE STUDY

Peter has been an occupational therapy assistant (OTA) for 5 years and has recently started a new job working at an inpatient rehabilitation facility. Peter's direct supervisor, Logan, is an occupational therapist (OT) who understands the scope of practice of an OTA and appears excited about developing a collaborative professional relationship. At Peter's 90-day new-hire review with Logan and the rehabilitation manager who is not an OT, Logan gives Peter excellent feedback commenting how quickly he has adapted to his new position. She mentioned that she was pleased with his interdisciplinary collaboration with physical therapy and noted that his contributions to the initial evaluations were valuable.

The next week Logan unexpectedly called out sick and the rehabilitation manager created the daily schedules for the OT practitioners. Peter noticed that he had been assigned three new evaluations to perform. When he brought this error to the rehabilitation manager's attention, she replied, "I have confidence in you. Logan said just the other day that you had great contributions to her evaluations. You can just do the entire evaluation and bill today. We will have Logan look at it tomorrow." Peter walked away from the conversation unsure of what to do next. He was concerned about his reputation and appearing competent. Peter knew that contributing to the initial evaluation was within his scope of practice but that the OT must be directly involved in and lead the initial evaluation.

Ethics is an integral part of every society and culture. It helps people understand the difference between what is right and wrong. Health care is a fast-paced, high-stakes environment; therefore, it is not surprising that health care professionals often face choices that raise ethical concerns. It is the responsibility of occupational therapy practitioners and every member of the interdisciplinary team to ensure that ethical care is a priority when these concerns arise. To provide ethical care, the practitioner must be familiar with ethical principles, overseeing agencies, common ethical issues, and strategies to foster an ethical culture in the workplace. This chapter will explore the components of ethics that impact the delivery of OT. Ethics is a challenging yet necessary topic for health care professionals because it affects the lives of clients. As an OTA, you are expected to have the foundational skills and knowledge to maintain high standards of responsible, ethical practice.

PRINCIPLES

When ethical issues arise, it can be difficult to know where to begin. Ethics education is often driven by principles; therefore, most people will use a principle-based approach to address a situation. Ethical principles are normative standards that are derived from common morality that can be applied to all situations. As an OTA, it is important that you have an understanding of some of these principles, as they will guide your thinking through different ethical issues and help you justify your subsequent actions (Limentani, 1999). In this section, we will explore the principles of beneficence, nonmaleficence, autonomy, justice, veracity, and fidelity. You must understand that these principles are not rigid and that they do not exist in a hierarchical formula. No one principle supersedes another—rather, they should be balanced. Occasionally, these principles may contradict each other, making it necessary to evaluate them in context to reach the optimum outcome. In addition to the principles, Beauchamp and Childress (2013) suggest that "experience and sound judgment are indispensable allies" (p. 395) when analyzing an ethical concern. We must also rely on our professional integrity. Professional integrity is the practice of consistently acting in an honest manner while upholding the standards of the profession. In the example of the case study, Peter must address the ethical issue to maintain his professional integrity. The following principles are widely accepted within bioethics and can be applied to occupational therapy.

Beneficence and Nonmaleficence

The principle of beneficence includes all forms of action intended to benefit others. In addition to doing good, it includes preventing or removing harm (Beauchamp & Childress, 2013). OT practitioners frequently encounter opportunities to provide beneficent care to clients in the form of ethical treatment interventions, defending basic rights of clients, and helping clients improve quality of life. Nonmaleficence is the principle to do no harm. Both principles are often combined in the literature, yet there is a distinct difference. Beneficence requires action to prevent or remove harm and promote good, while nonmaleficence requires no action.

Beneficence and nonmaleficence can seem discordant in some scenarios. For example, an OTA practicing in an outpatient clinic is treating a client with increased tone in her right upper extremity after a cerebrovascular accident. The client consistently reports discomfort with passive range of motion which could be considered harmful. After a few sessions of tolerating the uncomfortable range of motion, the client now has enough range of motion to drink from an adapted cup during meals independently. Although the intervention caused the client discomfort and could have been considered harmful in the moment, the eventual outcome of being able to incorporate her right arm into feeding tasks is a beneficent outcome. You must always consider the entire scenario to guide ethical decision making.

Autonomy

The principle of autonomy connotes an individual's right to make informed choices. It is often referred to as the self-determination principle because it represents a person's ability to determine his or her care. In the United States health care system, autonomy has popularly become thought of as the overarching principle that health care professionals rely upon during ethical decision-making. One explanation for such significant value being placed on autonomy could be that our society previously functioned using an extreme paternalistic approach. In the paternalistic approach, health care providers made decisions without client input. Today's health care professionals need to work toward bringing these two principles together so that our health care system incorporates a shared decision-making approach where care providers and clients collaborate to determine optimal plan of care (Figure 10-1).

Occupational therapy practitioners are well versed in client-centered care and collaborative goal setting. It is also important to understand the principle of autonomy as it relates to consent for treatment, participation in research, and the right to decline interventions. Individuals who have decision-making capacity must be active participants in the conversations regarding potential benefits and harms of treatment. As care providers, we must respect a person's right to choose his or her care even if it means declining treatment we have determined would be beneficial.

The following example is helpful in illustrating the principle of autonomy and the shared decision-making model. An OT and OTA are working with a client who is deemed to have decision-making capacity in an acute hospital setting. The occupational therapy discharge recommendations are for the client to transfer to an inpatient rehabilitation hospital. In a paternalistic society, the client would not have voice in the discharge planning process because the therapist would "know what's best." In a strictly autonomy-driven environment, the client would be given all potential options for discharge settings based on the health care professional's assessment; however, the practitioner would not make a recommendation, allowing the client to choose based on his or her preferences. Clearly, using solely a paternalistic or autonomous approach falls short of providing best care. In a shared decision-making model, the OT practitioner would discuss discharge options with the client, creating a dialogue. The OT practitioner would explain the options and make a clear recommendation based on clinical expertise while also respecting the individual's autonomy by considering his or her perspective.

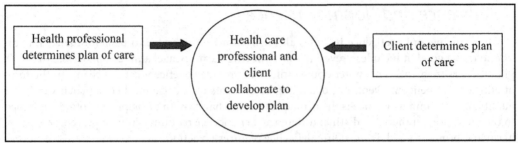

Figure 10-1. Shared decision-making continuum. (Adapted from Kon, A. A. [2010]. The shared decision-making continuum. *JAMA: The Journal of the American Medical Association, 304*, 903-904.)

Justice

The principle of justice includes both fair treatment of all people and the equitable distribution of resources. The United States is experiencing significant health care reform driven by the motivation to address the needs of all citizens, including those who are uninsured (see Chapter 1). The principle of justice is one that practitioners should aspire to enact; however, in practice there are limitations to providing equal care because of disparities that are inherent to our society. An OTA is not expected to transform policies to maintain this principle in practice. OTAs respect justice by advocating for clients from all backgrounds and socioeconomic classes. Respecting the principle of justice ensures impartial and righteous treatment of all clients.

For example, an OTA may identify a client's need for adaptive equipment or increased therapy; however, the ability to meet these needs is sometimes limited by the client's lack of insurance or personal financial limitations. In scenarios like this, OT practitioners should explore all alternative options. An OTA could research free care options for this client and connect him or her with local agencies that assist individuals ineligible for insurance.

Veracity

The principle of veracity is to be honest and truthful. According to Beauchamp and Childress (2013), "veracity in health care refers to accurate, timely, objective and comprehensive transmission of information" (p. 303). Truthfulness strengthens professional relationships with both colleagues and clients. Occupational therapy practitioners must accurately represent their credentials and communicate clearly. Occupational therapy practitioners should modify communication styles and teaching methods to meet each client's needs, taking into consideration cognitive abilities and education levels. In addition, to make certain that the client understands the communicated information, the OTA should use strategies such as the "teach-back method," where the client explains the information back to the care provider (Jager & Wynia, 2012).

For example, an OTA practicing in a skilled nursing facility develops an excellent rapport with a client and her family. Upon discharge from the skilled nursing facility, this client and family approach the OTA saying that they would like to privately hire an OT to evaluate and provide intervention in the home setting. The OTA in this example should clarify his credentials and explain the scope of practice of an OTA. It would violate the principle of veracity to continue the conversation without clarifying the OTA role.

Fidelity

The word *fidelity* is derived from the Latin *fidelis*, which means "faithful" or "loyal." This principle refers to a clinician's commitment to meeting a client's reasonable expectations (Purtilo & Doherty, 2011). To abide by this principle, the OTA should maintain a clear dialogue with the

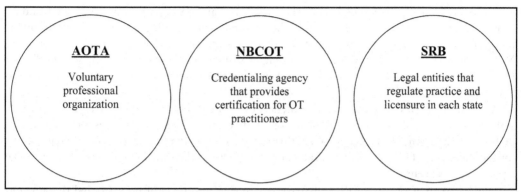

Figure 10-2. Occupational therapy governing entities.

client and interdisciplinary team. It is important to be aware of potential conflicts of interest and always attempt to resolve any misunderstandings about intentions.

For example, an OTA working in an outpatient clinic is scheduled to provide intervention for a close family friend. To maintain the principle of fidelity, the OTA should disclose this personal relationship to her supervisor and discuss potential conflicts of interest with the client.

PRACTICE STANDARDS

There are three separate entities that have established practice standards and enforcement procedures for OTs and OTAs. All occupational therapy practitioners should understand the roles and responsibilities of the AOTA, the National Board for Certification in Occupational Therapy (NBCOT), and the state regulatory boards (Figure 10-2).

The AOTA is the national professional organization of occupational therapy and is not a credentialing agency. Membership is strongly encouraged; however, it is voluntary. Within the AOTA, the Ethics Commission is one of the bodies of the Representative Assembly. The Ethics Commission is responsible for "writing, revising, and enforcing the *Occupational Therapy Code of Ethics and Ethics Standards* (2010)" (Slater, 2010, p. 39). The *Occupational Therapy Code of Ethics and Ethics Standards* is "a public statement of principles used to promote and maintain high standards within the profession" (AOTA, 2010a, p. 1). All members of the AOTA, including occupational therapists, occupational therapy assistants, and occupational therapy students, fall within the jurisdiction of the AOTA Ethics Commission and should be familiar with the practice standards.

The *Enforcement Procedures for the Occupational Therapy Code of Ethics and Ethics Standards* (AOTA, 2010b) was created to outline the process and jurisdiction of the Ethics Commission after an alleged violation is reported. It is important to note that the AOTA Ethics Commission can only review ethics complaints against occupational therapy practitioners who were members during the time of the alleged misconduct. You may access the *Occupational Therapy Code of Ethics and Ethics Standards* (AOTA, 2010a) and specific details on the process to file a complaint on www.aota.org.

The NBCOT is the credentialing agency that certifies OTAs and OTs (see Chapter 3). The NBCOT functions independently of the AOTA and is responsible for the initial certification examination, which most states require to practice. The NBCOT collaborates with the other agencies, such as the AOTA and the SRBs, by providing information on credentials, conduct, and certification issues. Once an OT is certified, he or she becomes a registered OT (OTR). Once an OTA is certified, he or she becomes a certified OTA (COTA). The NBCOT has its own practice standards outlined in the Candidate/Certificant Code of Conduct (NBCOT, 2014a), which includes sections on practice domains, professional conduct, supervision, and documentation.

Procedures for the enforcement of the NBCOT Candidate/Certificant Code of Conduct (NBCOT, 2014b) outlines the process for when an individual is alleged to have violated one or more of the principles. You can access the practice standards and enforcement procedures at NBCOT.org. The NBCOT has the jurisdiction to suspend or revoke a practitioner's COTA or OTR, so depending on the individual state's laws, this may impact an OT practitioner's ability to legally practice.

An SRB is a legal entity that has jurisdiction over practitioners licensed or regulated in that state. Each state has different requirements for practice and different procedures for filing a complaint. It is important for the occupational therapy practitioner to research the practice regulations for the state where he or she will be practicing. The SRB has the jurisdiction to restrict or revoke a practitioner's license.

The AOTA, NBCOT, and SRBs all strive to protect consumers of occupational therapy and maintain high standards of practice equally across the discipline. It is the responsibility of the clinician to ensure that he or she is lawfully and ethically providing occupational therapy services. A suspected violation of ethical principles may be reported to any or all of these entities; however, each entity has different jurisdictions and sanctions.

In the case study example, Peter's knowledge of practice standards allows him to easily identify that performing initial evaluations is outside of his scope of practice. His understanding of the roles of the AOTA, NBCOT, and his SRB help him identify potential resources for addressing the ethical issue.

Common Ethical Issues

Because of the changing health care system and the push to do more in less time, occupational therapy practitioners often face challenges in daily practice that can result in moral distress. Moral distress is the experience of knowing the ethically appropriate action but feeling powerless or constrained by external factors to implement it. It is important to be vigilant about identifying and addressing ethical issues to maintain high practice standards. Although at times it may be easier to ignore an ethical concern, as an OTA you are obligated to do what is best for your clients and the profession. In the case study, Peter knows that he cannot perform the initial evaluations without direct involvement of an OT; however, he is concerned that the rehab director may see this as incompetence. Many of the common ethical issues that occur in the clinical setting relate to three major areas, including productivity, supervision, and caseload competence.

Productivity, which is billing for a specific number of units, is the typical way in which OT practitioners are deemed to be meeting workplace expectations. It is the responsibility of the professional to know and adhere to ethical standards set forth by the AOTA, NBCOT, and your SRB. It is the professional duty of OTAs to ensure that while striving to meet the productivity standards of their workplace, ethical and legal standards are still being upheld. When an OTA feels that the productivity standards are unreasonable and unachievable in an ethical way, he or she must pursue further conversations with supervisors and administration. It is never acceptable to falsely bill for services that were not provided or not clinically appropriate, as this would be considered fraud and would violate ethical standards.

Supervision is an important part of professional development (see Chapter 7). Occupational therapy practitioners must be aware of the practice acts, regulations, and organizational expectations regarding supervision. Every OTA should have a relationship with an OT in his or her work setting. It can be easy to let supervision fall below standards, especially when you are working in a fast-paced environment with high client volume and complexity. Although it is important to put client needs first, to ensure that ethical and legal care is consistently being provided, supervision by an OT needs to be a priority. As an OTA, you should be familiar with the professional expectations for supervision and ensure that you are meeting them.

Caseload competence can be a difficult issue to address because it puts the OTA or OT in a vulnerable position. Caseload competence includes having both the knowledge to treat certain populations and the ability to manage a certain number of clients in a workday. There is a broad range of issues related to caseload that can bring about moral distress. An OT practitioner should demonstrate competence with various diagnoses and impairments before providing intervention. A practitioner should maintain open communication with supervisors to determine continuing education needs. In addition, it is important to ensure that your expected caseload matches your ability to efficiently and effectively provide high-quality occupational therapy. Sometimes, employees can feel uncomfortable raising issues about caseload because they fear that doing so may make them appear incompetent. It is necessary to address these issues to maintain high practice standards for occupational therapy. Effective supervisors will work with you to achieve competence.

Often in ethical dilemmas, one must act with moral courage. Moral courage is the willingness to uphold moral and ethical values despite the risk of criticism or negative feedback. When an ethical issue or dilemma is identified, a decision-making framework can be helpful to determine how to proceed. There are many different decision-making frameworks available in the literature. Figure 10-3 is a suggested model to use when OT practitioners encounter ethical issues in practice.

The decision-making framework starts with identifying an ethical issue. Rather than acting immediately, one should think through a deliberate process. Once the issue is identified, one should gather relevant information and facts. After obtaining all of the facts, you should identify potential resources. These resources may include colleagues, supervisors, policies, administrators, and professional organizations. Next, you need to evaluate your options, which could include initiating a conversation with the alleged violator, bringing your concerns to supervisors, or filing a formal complaint with the AOTA, NBCOT, or an SRB. Once you have weighed the various options considering potential outcomes, you should choose your best option and act. The process does not end there because it is important to reflect on your actions and the outcome. Using this decision-making framework will ensure a thoughtful response and avoid reactive or impulsive actions.

In the case study, Peter identifies the ethical issue as a supervisor delegating responsibilities to him that are outside his scope of practice. He then gathers the facts and organizes the relevant information. He identifies his resources at the AOTA, Medicare, and SRB, which all clearly indicate that evaluation is not within the scope of practice for an OTA. Peter considers his options: he can ignore the issue and perform the evaluations as directed, he can bring copies of these documents to his rehabilitation manager, or he can contact his SRB and file a formal complaint against the rehabilitation manager. Peter decides that he will bring copies of the state regulations to the rehabilitation manager and discuss the concern again. This time, the rehabilitation manager apologizes for her mistake, stating that she misunderstood the regulations and would remove the initial evaluations from Peter's caseload. As Peter reflected on his actions, he was proud that he had the moral courage to approach the supervisor and to maintain the high standards of the occupational therapy profession.

FOSTERING AN ETHICAL CULTURE

Health care is a dynamic and complex environment where professionals confront complex ethical issues each day. This chapter has focused on principles, common ethical issues, and strategies to address ethical issues, but what we have not discussed yet is how to foster an ethical culture to prevent these issues from occurring. Addressing each individual ethics issue as it occurs is inadequate. We must create underlying systems and a culture that support the prevention of ethical issues. Walker (1993) describes ethics as not a question of mastering code-like theories and law-like principles—rather, she suggests that health care professionals are architects of moral space. OT practitioners can shape the moral space of their environment in many ways, including

Figure 10-3. Ethical decision-making framework.

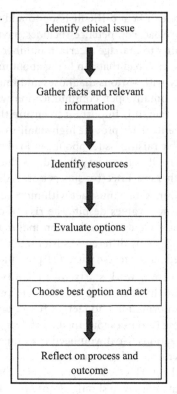

identifying themes and triggers, maintaining high professional standards, placing value on effective communication, implementing ethics rounds, or supporting involvement in ethics committees.

Identifying Common Themes and Triggers

Taking the time to review and analyze past ethical issues will begin to shed light on trends and common triggers of ethical conflict (Epstein, 2012). Each setting and department will have its own unique triggers; therefore, it is important for the OT practitioner to frequently assess the needs of his or her work environment. Potential triggers could include increased wait times for clients, inconsistent care providers, inadequate documentation, lack of team consensus, or poor communication between team members. Once a trend or trigger is identified, specific interventions can be developed to minimize future conflicts. Preventative ethics is a strategy of implementing system-based changes to thwart common ethical issues from arising. It involves analyzing causes and factors of past ethical issues. It will be impossible to eliminate all ethical issues because of the dynamic nature of health care; however, learning from past events is key to early recognition and limiting the escalation of future conflicts.

Maintaining High Professional Standards

You must represent yourself and occupational therapy by maintaining the highest professional standards. This includes not only having strong knowledge about the scope of practice within the state in which you are licensed, but also having a foundational understanding of the ethical expectations of a health care professional as set forth by the employer, the AOTA, NBCOT, and SRB. These entities aim to maintain high standards to protect the consumer and the reputation of the discipline.

Communication

Effective communication strategies have been highlighted in Chapter 9; however, it is important to emphasize that communication is a key component to fostering an ethical culture. The aspects of communication that are most pertinent to ethics are as follows:

- Making expectations clear
- Maintaining confidentiality
- Communicating clearly, truthfully, and in a timely manner
- Ensuring that clients truly understand treatment before providing informed consent
- Safeguarding individuals who wish to raise ethical concerns from harassment or punitive repercussions

An OTA should work closely with the OT and interdisciplinary team to improve communication that will result in effective ethical care of clients.

Ethics Rounds

Developing a forum for team members to openly and honestly reflect on ethical issues can have a powerful impact on fostering an ethical culture. Ethics rounds are most effective when an interdisciplinary team is present but can also focus on issues unique to the OT profession. Successful ethics rounds can be topic based or on a specific case. By implementing an ethics rounds schedule, the OT practitioner is making a clear statement that ethics is a priority in his or her practice and modeling behavior for other team members.

Committee Involvement

Most hospitals and health care settings are required to have ethics committees. Occupational therapy practitioners can provide distinct contributions to these discussions because of expertise in client-centered practice, collaborative goal setting, and meaningful participation. An OTA should explore options within his or her work setting and community to represent the discipline of OT in these discussions. OTA managers should encourage staff to dedicate time to these committees.

CONCLUSION

This chapter discussed ethical principles as an approach to understanding ethical issues that arise in practice. We focused on beneficence, nonmaleficence, autonomy, justice, veracity, and fidelity, understanding that there is no hierarchy to these principles, yet they should all be considered and balanced when examining a situation. Next, we looked at the agencies that are involved in occupational therapy practice, including the AOTA, NBCOT, and the SRB. Each of these agencies has different processes for responding to alleged ethical violations, and it is the responsibility of practitioners to know the practice standards and regulations for the state that they are practicing in. We then went on to look at common ethical issues and an example of a decision-making framework to guide your thinking. Lastly, we discussed strategies for fostering an ethical culture and preventative ethics. As you have hopefully come to understand, ethics is a critical component of providing high-quality occupational therapy services to clients. Practitioners must maintain their individual moral character and be informed about practice standards. All OTAs will face ethical issues in their careers, and this chapter provides you with the skills to identify and address them.

Suggested Websites

- American Occupational Therapy Association ethics: www.aota.org
- National Board for Certification in Occupational Therapy professional conduct: http://www.nbcot.org/professional-conduct
- The Hastings Center: www.thehastingscenter.org
- Presidential Commission for the Study of Bioethical Issues: www.bioethics.gov

Review Questions

1. Which ethical principle addresses an individual's right to make informed choices?
   a. Beneficence
   b. Justice
   c. Autonomy
   d. Moral courage

2. Which of the following statements best describes shared decision making?
   a. The care provider tells the client what to do.
   b. The client instructs the care provider on what to do.
   c. The client and care provider collaborate to determine the optimal plan of care.
   d. The client and care provider ask a third party to determine optimal plan of care.

3. The ethical principle of justice is:
   a. Fair treatment of all people and the equitable distribution of resources
   b. To do no harm
   c. Autonomy
   d. Consistently acting in an honest manner while upholding professional standards

4. Which of the following is the ethical principle to do no harm?
   a. Beneficence
   b. Fidelity
   c. Nonmaleficence
   d. Moral courage

5. Which of the following statements is true about the AOTA Ethics Commission?
   a. It has jurisdiction over all OTs and OTAs.
   b. It is responsible for licensing OTs and OTAs.
   c. It can revoke license to practice.
   d. It is responsible for writing, revising, and enforcing the *Occupational Therapy Code of Ethics and Ethics Standards*.

6. What organization(s) have ethical oversight of the occupational therapy profession?

    a. AOTA

    b. NBCOT

    c. SRBs

    d. All of the above

7. If an OTA identifies an ethical concern with a colleague's billing, the OTA should:

    a. Ignore it in order to avoid embarrassing the colleague

    b. Immediately file a formal complaint with the AOTA

    c. Implement a decision-making framework before acting

    d. Immediately file a formal complaint with the SRB

8. Which of the following best describes moral courage?

    a. Upholding moral and ethical values despite the risk of criticism

    b. Knowing the ethically appropriate action to take, but feeling powerless

    c. Respecting an individual's right to make an informed decision

    d. Ignoring ethical principles because of fear or retaliation

9. Why is it important to analyze trends of ethical issues in your work setting?

    a. To place blame on practitioners who consistently raise issues

    b. To implement strategies aimed at eliminating triggers and preventing future issues

    c. To maintain the principle of autonomy

    d. To demonstrate which practitioners are interested in ethics

10. How can an OTA foster an ethical culture in the workplace?

    a. By creating ethics rounds

    b. By maintaining confidentiality

    c. By modeling best practice

    d. All of the above

REFERENCES

American Occupational Therapy Association. (2010a). Occupational Therapy Code of Ethics and Ethics Standards. *American Journal of Occupational Therapy, 64*(6 Suppl.), S17–S26.

American Occupational Therapy Association. (2010b). Enforcement Procedures for the Occupational Therapy Code of Ethics and Ethics Standards. *American Journal of Occupational Therapy, 64*(6 Suppl.), S4-S16.

Beauchamp, T. L., & Childress, J. F. (2013). *Principles of biomedical ethics* (7th ed.). New York: Oxford University Press.

Epstein, E. G. (2012). Ethics in critical care: Preventative ethics in the intensive care unit. *AACN Advanced Critical Care, 23,* 214-224.

Jager, A. J., & Wynia, M. K. (2012). Who gets a teach-back? Patient-reported incidence of experiencing a teach-back. *Journal of Health Communication: International Perspectives, 17,* 294-302.

Limentani, A. (1999). The role of ethical principles in health care and the implications for ethical codes. *Journal of Medical Ethics, 25,* 394-398.

National Board for Certification in Occupational Therapy. (2014a). *NBCOT candidate/certificant code of conduct.* Retrieved from http://www.nbcot.org/certificant-code-of-conduct

National Board for Certification in Occupational Therapy. (2014b). *Procedures for the enforcement of the NBCOT candidate/certificant code of conduct.* Retrieved from http://www.nbcot.org/procedures-for-enforcement

Purtilo, R. B., & Doherty, R. F. (2011). *Ethical dimensions in the health professions* (5th ed.). St. Louis, MO: Elsevier Saunders.

Slater, D. Y. (2010). Reference guide to the occupational therapy code of ethics and ethics standards. Bethesda, MD: AOTA Press.

Walker, M. U. (1993). Keeping moral spaces open: New images of ethics consulting. *The Hastings Center Report, 23,* 33-40.

11

The Importance of Scholarship and Scholarly Practice for the OTA

Linda Niemeyer, OT, PhD

ACOTE Standards explored in this chapter:

- B.8.0. Scholarship. Promotion of scholarly endeavors will serve to describe and interpret the scope of the profession, establish new knowledge, and interpret and apply this knowledge to practice. The program must facilitate development of the performance criteria listed below. The student will be able to:

- B.8.1. Articulate the importance of how scholarly activities contribute to the development of a body of knowledge relevant to the profession of occupational therapy.

- B.8.2. Effectively locate, understand, critique, and evaluate information, including the quality of evidence.

- B.8.3. Use scholarly literature to make evidence-based decisions.

- B.8.7. Participate in scholarly activities that evaluate professional practice, service delivery, and/or professional issues (e.g., Scholarship of Integration, Scholarship of Application, Scholarship of Teaching and Learning).

KEY VOCABULARY

Scholarship: Research activities designed to build the knowledge base of occupational therapy to further advance practice and teaching.

Scholarly practice: Evidence-based practice; using the knowledge base of the profession in occupational therapy practice and teaching.

Jacobs K, ed.
Management and Administration for the OTA:
Leadership and Application Skills (pp 143-156).
© 2016 Taylor & Francis Group.

Case Study #1, Part 1

An occupational therapist (OT) has developed a meal preparation group as part of the inpatient rehabilitation program at a large teaching hospital (Littleton, 2013). The group serves individuals with a range of cognitive and/or physical deficits. The aim of the intervention is to "promote socialization, confidence, and independent living skills" (Littleton, 2013, p. 7). Let's consider the possibility that because of growing enthusiasm for this program, you have been brought in to share the workload with the OT. Moreover, let's suppose that the OT has been charged by hospital administration to gather data in a study designed to demonstrate that the intervention is helping participants to meet rehabilitation goals. You are to assist with this study.

Quantitative research: Use of the scientific method to gather data that can be expressed numerically and analyzed statistically to describe population characteristics and/or determine the relationship between one or more independent and dependent variables.

Qualitative research: Exploratory gathering of in-depth, detailed descriptions of problems or conditions from the point of view of the group or individual experiencing them to discover themes and their interrelationships or linkages.

Independent variable: A factor in research such as an intervention that can be manipulated by the investigator; also, a stable characteristic of individuals by which they can be grouped.

Dependent variable: One or more clinical findings, behaviors, personal attributes, or internal experiences that are measured in research; the dependent variable might be hypothesized to change as the result of the independent variable or to differ among independent variable groupings.

Rigor: Close adherence to experimental research methodology; in broader usage, embedding of sound principles and practices—agreed upon by the scientific community—into each step of the quantitative or qualitative research process in order to ensure trustworthiness of results.

Introduction: The Evolving Need for Scholarship

At the turn of the millennium, Holm (2000) in her Eleanor Clarke Slagle Lecture reflected on the challenges that would be facing occupational therapy practitioners in the next century. Beginning in the mid-1970s, occupational therapy practitioners had encountered new developments in health care delivery and reimbursement, including managed care, prospective payment, capitation, and changes in staffing ratios, which greatly affected the way services were provided (see Chapter 1). Moreover, there was an increasing demand for justifying practice patterns via research-based evidence demonstrating that occupational therapy interventions resulted in improved client outcomes. The demand was not only that research evidence should demonstrate positive outcomes, but also that it should provide enough information about what was done in the intervention, and how it was done, so that others could replicate it with comparable clients and achieve similar outcomes.

Indeed, this new emphasis on justifying occupational therapy practice patterns was reflected in an influx of published evidence. On the surface, this was encouraging news, but regrettably several problems were recognized. First, the quantity of the published evidence that practitioners would need to sift through was daunting. Second, Holm (2000) analyzed the quality of the evidence in articles published by the *Occupational Therapy Journal of Research* between 1995 and 1999 and found that more than 50% provided the weakest evidence in the form of descriptive studies or the opinions of experts, while barely 8% represented what the author would consider the strongest evidence in the form of true experimental studies. Third, when occupational therapy practice is based on limited or insufficient evidence, this undoubtedly creates an ethical dilemma. If the safety and well-being of recipients of OT services is to be ensured, knowledge derived from current research must be incorporated into clinical practice. Occupational therapy academicians and practitioners tackled this challenge by developing a new conceptual framework for scholarship and scholarly practice.

SCHOLARLY ENDEAVORS AND THEIR CONTRIBUTION TO THE OCCUPATIONAL THERAPY BODY OF KNOWLEDGE

There are several types of scholarly endeavors identified in the occupational therapy literature that can be conceived of as being separate yet interrelated. The new conceptual framework for scholarship was outlined in a 2009 American Occupational Therapy Association (AOTA) position paper. First, the authors distinguished between scholarly practice and scholarship. Scholarly practice, otherwise known as evidence-based practice, was defined as "using the knowledge base of the profession or discipline in one's practice" and in teaching (AOTA, 2009, p. 790). On the other hand, scholarship was equated with activities designed to build the knowledge base and further advance the practice and teaching of occupational therapy; these activities also came under the heading of research. With regard to the evidence gained through scholarly practice and scholarship, the authors concluded, "All occupational therapists and occupational therapy assistants, regardless of their individual practice roles, have the professional responsibility to not only use that evidence to inform their professional decision making but also to generate new evidence through independent or collaborative research, or both" (AOTA, 2009, p. 793).

Tickle-Degnan (1999) described the role of evidence-based practice in occupational therapy by characterizing it as a set of organizing and evaluating tools "designed to integrate research study evidence into the clinical reasoning process" to "help the practitioner select the best assessments and intervention procedures from an array of possibilities" (p. 537) and achieve the best possible outcomes. According to the classic definition of evidence-based practice, the occupational therapy practitioner is asked to integrate his or her own internal clinical expertise with the best available relevant external systematic research to inform practice decisions (Kielhofner, 2006; Law & MacDermid, 2008; Taylor, 2007). The recommended procedure for conducting an evidence-based practice inquiry will be discussed later in this chapter. This process calls for a certain amount of flexibility in the practitioner's willingness to modify assessment or intervention in response to the new knowledge gained. The rewards of improved competency in both research skills and clinical practice are much valued by stakeholders, particularly those whose primary focus is consumer protection and judicious use of resources (Christiansen & Lou, 2001; Kielhofner, 2006).

Fortunately, ongoing debate and discussion has led to some evolution regarding implementation of evidence-based practice, which has enhanced its applicability to occupational therapy (Christiansen & Lou, 2001; Kielhofner, 2006; Law & MacDermid, 2008). Most notable is the acknowledgment of the importance of the values, needs, and preferences of the client and his or her family. In this adapted format, the occupational therapy practitioner bases clinical decisions on his or her own expertise and the best evidence available while also consulting with the client and family to help determine the most suitable option. The client's perspective is thus taken into account; the evidence and its meaning are translated into user-friendly terms, and choices are made based on client-practitioner collaboration (Dijkers, Murphy, & Krellman, 2012; Tickle-Degnan, 1999). In this way, evidence-based practice becomes better suited to the client-centered values and philosophy of occupational therapy.

Let us now turn our attention from scholarly practice, or evidence-based practice, to an expanded conception of scholarship. Haertlein and Coppard (2003), as well as the AOTA (2009),

CASE STUDY #1, PART 2

The first 2 weeks in your new position are spent observing and participating in the meal preparation program. During this time, the OT explains the role of scholarship in the inception of the program and its continued development.

The OT describes how scholarly practice, or evidence-based practice, played a key role in the design of the current program. Together, you review and evaluate the knowledge base, as represented in the published literature, which served as the basis for the initial justification and design of the program. You note that some of the articles provided guiding theoretical principles, while in others the authors portrayed occupational therapy interventions that included a cooking group and the information they gathered about clients' perceptions of the group using surveys. The populations in these studies included individuals recovering from burns and clients in a stroke rehabilitation program.

You discuss with the OT how the mix of participants in the current program is a much broader representation of rehabilitation clients than presented in the literature. During the 2 weeks, you worked with four clients who were recovering from stroke, one who was post coronary artery bypass surgery, one who had a brain tumor, one who was dealing with pulmonary problems, two with spinal injuries, two with cognitive deficits, and an amputee. These participants exhibited both high and low levels of physical and cognitive function. In addition, accepted practice is to evaluate the effectiveness of the program in terms of the clients' subjective perceptions of value and benefit. If the goal of the current program is to improve independent living skills, shouldn't improvement in actual function be recorded objectively before, during, and after the program and following discharge from the facility?

Based on this discussion, you realize that clearly there are gaps in the available knowledge for this type of program in the published literature. The current study being planned by the OT is an opportunity for scholarship. You will be able to contribute to a research activity that will help fill in the gaps and build the knowledge base of occupational therapy so as to further advance practice and teaching.

described four dimensions of scholarship, which are based on the seminal work of American educator Earnest L. Boyer:

1. *The scholarship of discovery.* Conducting original scientific research; this type of scholarship contributes to the growing knowledge base of occupational therapy.

2. *The scholarship of integration.* Seeking new insights from existing original research, both within occupational therapy and across disciplines, by integrating, interpreting, and synthesizing in a search for new patterns of connection; this type of scholarship contributes to the formation of new perspectives and theories in occupational therapy.

3. *The scholarship of application.* Forging a link between theory and practice and between academia and service provision; this type of scholarship contributes to the use of knowledge and insights gained from the scholarship of discovery and integration to address societal problems, occupational therapy assessments or interventions, or classroom teaching of clients or occupational therapy practitioners in a practical way.

4. *The scholarship of teaching and learning.* Systematic study based on the recognition of the complementary nature of teaching and learning; this type of scholarship contributes to the knowledge base needed for high-quality teaching of occupational therapy students and for public sharing of the knowledge of the profession.

The types of scholarly endeavors that were discussed in this section are reviewed in Figure 11-1. Ongoing work by occupational therapy academicians and practitioners has led to the understanding that building of the occupational therapy body of knowledge via scholarly practice and

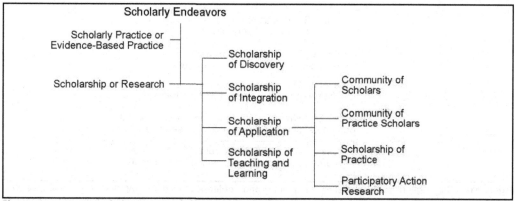

Figure 11-1. An expanded conception of scholarship as the means for building occupational therapy body of knowledge. (Reprinted with permission from Jacobs, K., MacRae, N., & Sladyk, K. [2014]. *Occupational therapy essentials for clinical competence* [2nd ed.]. Thorofare, NJ: SLACK Incorporated; 583.)

scholarship entails an ongoing dialog that brings together occupational therapy theoretical concepts, empirical research to verify those concepts, and real-world application of those concepts by means of clinical practice and active collaboration with the community. Any occupational therapy practitioner, regardless of his or her role in the profession, thus has the opportunity to help fulfill the ethical responsibility to contribute to the generation of knowledge that leads to steady progression of the profession of occupational therapy.

THE NATURE AND QUALITY OF EVIDENCE

The core of any scholarly endeavor, including scholarly practice (or evidence-based practice) and scholarship (or research), is the ability to judge the quality of evidence. Basically, quality of evidence might be conceived of as the degree of confidence an occupational therapy practitioner or academician can have in the trustworthiness, accuracy, relevance, and usefulness of information from a published research approach for making practice decisions. An understanding of the quality of evidence is also of critical importance for designing the best possible research approach to substantiate occupational therapy theory or practice methodology. The traditional guideline for judging the quality of evidence was largely established in evidence-based medicine as a single hierarchical system based on study categories and usually termed *levels of evidence* (Law & MacDermid, 2008; Sackett, Rosenberg, Gray, Haynes, & Richardson, 1996; Taylor, 2007). This hierarchical system has been widely adopted, sometimes with minor modifications and will be found in AOTA Web-based materials (AOTA, n.d.a, n.d.b). It can be visualized as a simple two-dimensional pyramid, as seen in Figure 11-2, with the weakest or lowest-quality sources of evidence at the bottom and the strongest or highest-quality sources of evidence at the apex.

Experimental research, particularly the randomized controlled trial, is thus considered to be the highest level of evidence. At the core of any experimental design is the intent to establish, by means of statistical tests, the probability that an intervention—called the *independent variable*—caused change in one or more clinical findings—called the *dependent variable(s)*—in a population of interest (Kielhofner, 2006). In classical evidence-based medicine, experimental studies, or clinical trials, the independent variable is a medication, clinical procedure, or treatment and investigators select the dependent variable(s) based on clinical relevance. True experiments are *prospective*, meaning that data from measurement of the dependent variable(s) are gathered both prior to and after the intervention and are used to determine the degree to which the intervention led to change. This is in

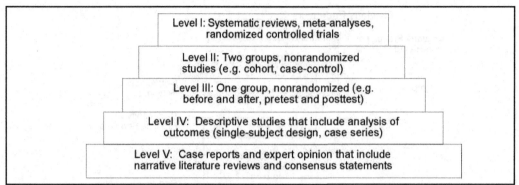

Figure 11-2. The single hierarchical system for categorization of levels of evidence (AOTA, 2012) shown as a two-dimensional pyramid with the weakest sources of evidence at the base and the strongest sources of evidence at the apex. (Reprinted with permission from Jacobs, K., MacRae, N., & Sladyk, K. [2014]. *Occupational therapy essentials for clinical competence* [2nd ed.]. Thorofare, NJ: SLACK Incorporated; 583.)

contrast to retrospective research, wherein data that are collected can refer to both current and past events, phenomena, or clinical findings. Individuals chosen to participate in experimental research ideally can be shown to be representative of a much larger population of individuals based on a close approximation of relevant characteristics such as age, gender, education, diagnosis, or impairment.

Experimental research extends beyond classical applications, particularly in studies conducted by occupational therapy and other health professionals. The independent variable can be a treatment, and it also can be a prevention or screening protocol, a form of diagnostic testing, a health care setting, or an educational program. Researchers may select a relevant physical or physiological clinical finding, such as heart rate, breathing patterns, specific laboratory test results, joint range of motion, or muscle strength, as a dependent variable. They may also consider clinical findings that are behaviors or personal attributes, particularly those of importance to clients and their families, caregivers, teachers, or employers, because they are related to functioning in one or more aspects of everyday life. A behavior might be chosen as a dependent variable because it is considered inappropriate, disturbing, or disruptive. A selected personal attribute might be the ability to process sensory information or to perform activities of daily living or a skill such as handwriting. Finally, the dependent variable can be an internal experience such as perceived pain or quality of life.

The three key characteristics of true experimental studies, which are also chief considerations for establishing levels of evidence in experimental research, are control, randomization, and blinding. *Control* customarily describes the presence of a control group in which participants receive no intervention or engage in neutral activity unrelated to the intervention. Participants can also be assigned to a comparison group in which they receive an alternate intervention. The inclusion of control groups helps support the scientific conclusion that any notable differences in the dependent variable between groups can be attributed to the intervention and not to some other, unidentified causal factor. One can conceive of another aspect of control, which is the assurance that all individuals within each experimental group are treated identically. Often the term *fidelity* is used to indicate that the independent variable is administered exactly as planned and is true to the underlying theory of the intervention.

Randomization means that assignment of participants to an intervention or control group is made using a statistical technique, such as a random number table, so that each participant has an equal likelihood of being a member of any group. This means that the investigators, the individuals providing the intervention, or the study participants in no way directly influence assignment to group. If randomization is properly carried out, there is a high likelihood that the characteristics of participants in each group will be similar. Blinding refers to a process of concealing knowledge of which participant in the experimental population is receiving what intervention or control condition; it can be extended to participants, individuals engaged in providing an intervention or recording dependent variables, or individuals analyzing data from the study. The purpose of blinding is to prevent conscious or unconscious expectations from coloring a participant's response to an intervention, an intervention provider's response to the participant, or the recording or analysis of information by members of the research team. Blinding is not always possible for several practical reasons. For example, it might not be feasible to conceal from a practitioner or participant the nature of the intervention that is being administered.

Though the randomized controlled clinical trial has been extolled as the most robust method for providing evidence linking health care to end results, conducting this type of experimental research is not always logically feasible for the clinical setting (Ottenbacher & Hinderer, 2001). Clinical trials are demanding of available resources. For example, they call for a large number of participants who have similar characteristics and for highly controlled experimental conditions. Moreover, ethical considerations can arise when participants who are randomly assigned to a control condition receive no intervention.

Outcome research designs, often termed quasi-experimental, represent viable alternatives that, if conducted with sufficient attention to detail, can provide a quantitative estimate of the impact of an intervention or of certain participant characteristics on one or more dependent variables (Cooper, Hedges, & Valentine, 2009; Kielhofner, 2006; Wholey, Hatry, & Newcomer, 2010). Outcome studies are called quasi-experimental because, for practical or ethical reasons, they lack some or all of the features of true experimental studies, namely prospective design, a control group, randomization, and blinding. However, as a method of determining the effectiveness of a program, outcome research can address important clinical findings, the internal experiences of recipients of care, a broad array of health care delivery factors, and consumer preferences (Wholey et al., 2010).

Qualitative research is a non-experimental approach that resonates well with the holistic and client-centered worldview, as well as the core concerns, assumptions, and values, of occupational therapy (Cook, 2001; Kielhofner, 1982a, 2006; Merrill, 1985). It constitutes a naturalistic method of scientific inquiry that is fundamentally exploratory and subjective and whose primary aim is to gather in-depth, detailed descriptions of a phenomenon of interest, such as a problem or condition, from the point of view of the group or individual experiencing it. Inquiry does not stop at the level of describing the problem or condition, but seeks to interpret each phenomenon in light of physical, social, economic, regulatory, and cultural contexts as well as personal viewpoints, meanings, and perceptions (Kielhofner, 1982b, 2006; Merrill, 1985; Papadimitriou, Magasi, & Frank, 2012). Quantitative experimental and outcome research approaches cannot adequately capture these interwoven and sometimes elusive complexities for a number of reasons (Kielhofner, 1982b; Merrill, 1985). First, when conducting quantitative research, investigators characteristically test hypotheses based on existing theories. Second, quantitative investigators use standardized methods of data collection and numerical analysis to yield findings on pre-established variables. Third, the quantitative discovery process is linear, proceeding from the definition of a research problem through a sequence of steps and concluding with reporting of findings and often generation of new research questions.

However, in qualitative approaches, the discovery process is cyclical and open-ended, driven by the perspectives of the participants and not of the researchers (Cook, 2001). Methodology, concepts, and theory develop gradually as the research progresses and are derived as the accumulated data and interpretations lend structure and focus (Kielhofner, 1982b, 2006; Merrill, 1985). Methods of data collection include in-depth unstructured or semi-structured interviews, focus groups, participant or field observation, and review of pertinent records and other documents (Cook, 2001; Mack, Woodsong, MacQueen, Guest, & Namey, 2005). Data are documented via written notes, photographs, audio recordings, and video recordings. The goal of analysis and interpretation is to reduce data to recurring patterns of conceptual categories and themes via a painstaking process of review. As meaning and significance emerge, a model is constructed depicting interrelationships or linkages (Wholey et al., 2010).

Case Study #2

During the third week of hands-on experience with the meal preparation group, the OT explains about the plan for the current study. Some aspects of the published research will be replicated, while some unique methodology will be added to fit the setting and participants for the program. This is to be a prospective quasi-experimental or outcome study. The design was chosen because, for practical and ethical reasons, at this time it is not feasible to assign participants randomly to intervention and control groups.

The occupational therapy intervention provided during the meal preparation group is the independent variable. For the dependent variables, the OT would like to gather participants' perceptions of the value and benefit of the program using a survey as well as information about actual function in meal preparation.

Both quantitative and qualitative data will be collected. The survey includes three questions that are rated on a 5-point scale plus two open-ended questions. Using a check sheet, the observer will numerically rate degree of mastery of selected kitchen tasks, with or without adaptation. These data will be gathered during and after each program session. Following discharge from the facility, the survey will be administered one more time via telephone. The telephone interviewer will also ask open-ended questions about the participant's socialization, confidence, and functional performance in the kitchen at home, which will provide additional qualitative information.

One other classification of nonexperimental research is worth mentioning. In longitudinal research, data are collected on selected characteristics or dependent variables in a population of interest at multiple points in time, possibly over months or years. Data might also be collected on interventions or other aspects of health care received by the population, and groups who did or did not receive this care are compared. There is no investigator manipulation; the primary objective is to detect numerical patterns of stability and change that develop over time and that allow investigators to make statistical inferences regarding how and why change did or did not take place (Kielhofner, 2006). Some sources use the term *cohort designs* for this type of research (Law et al., 1998a).

Understanding Validity

Another important hallmark of quality is research validity, which is a core issue for all scientific inquiry, regardless of design (Kielhofner, 1982b). Research validity serves as an indication of the degree to which research methods and findings are sound in that they reflect actual phenomena in the world and are not distorted by inaccuracies in conceptual or theoretical foundations, design, measurement, or analysis. Another term for research validity is *rigor*, or trustworthiness. In traditional usage, rigor refers to close adherence to experimental research methodology; in broader usage, rigor can be described as embedding sound principles and practices—agreed upon by the scientific community—into each step of a quantitative or qualitative research process in order to ensure trustworthiness of results (Kielhofner, 2006).

Table 11-1 puts forth a well-developed conceptual model, first developed by Guba (1981), and Krefting (1991), which identifies four key criteria for evaluating research validity or trustworthiness that can be applied to both the quantitative and qualitative perspectives. The terminology used reflects the distinct philosophical, conceptual, and methodological differences of these two perspectives. However, it should be kept in mind that one approach can be used to complement and corroborate the other and thereby extend the scope of inquiry (Mortenson & Oliffe, 2009).

TABLE 11-1

FOUR CRITERIA FOR EVALUATING THE TRUSTWORTHINESS OF RESEARCH FROM BOTH THE QUANTITATIVE AND QUALITATIVE PERSPECTIVES

CRITERION	QUALITATIVE RESEARCH PERSPECTIVE	QUANTITATIVE RESEARCH PERSPECTIVE
Truth value: the level of confidence in the veracity of research findings that the investigators were able to establish, given the study's design, subjects or informants, and context.	Credibility: the degree of accuracy in preserving and representing the holistic situation and participants being studied, as well as in describing and interpreting the experiences of participants in a way that is immediately recognizable by these individuals.	Internal validity: the extent to which a causal connection can be established between an intervention, or independent variable, and one or more outcomes, or dependent variables; identification and ruling out of factors other than the independent variable that could influence or mask the research findings.
Applicability: the extent to which the findings of a research study can be applied to other contexts, settings, and groups or generalized to larger populations.	Transferability: the level of representativeness of the informants or participants for the particular group being studied, such that other program providers can apply the findings to their context.	External validity: the extent to which research findings can be generalized or applied beyond the groups or contexts specific to the study.
Consistency: the degree to which the research findings are reproducible, given that the study is duplicated with the same participants and setting or context.	Dependability: the extent to which the uniqueness or repeatability of a study has been established by means of thorough and exact description of the methods of data gathering, analysis, and interpretation, as well as by use of methods to replicate and confirm the accuracy of this information.	Reliability: the extent to which an experimental or outcome study would yield the same result if repeated independently; the extent to which a measurement used in a study would produce the same results with different raters or repeat administration over time.
Neutrality: the level of freedom from bias, meaning that research findings are not influenced by the personal motivations or perspectives of the investigators but are the sole function of the conditions of the study.	Confirmability: the degree of understanding of how and why decisions were made in a study, such that another researcher would arrive at comparable conclusions given the same data and research context, established using an external and/or internal auditing process to review data, findings, interpretations, and recommendations.	Objectivity: the extent to which judgments made and data recorded during the research process are based solely on observed phenomena without the influence of personal agendas, emotions, prejudices, assumptions, or predispositions.

Adapted from Guba, E. G. (1981). ERIC/ECTJ annual review paper: Criteria for assessing the trustworthiness of naturalistic inquiries. *Educational Communication and Technology Journal, 29*(2), 75-91; Krefting, L. (1991). Rigor in qualitative research: The assessment of trustworthiness. *American Journal of Occupational Therapy, 45*(3), 214-222; and Wholey, J. S., Hatry, H. P., & Newcomer, K. E. (2010). *Handbook of practical program evaluation* (3rd ed.). San Francisco: John Wiley & Sons. (Reprinted from Jacobs, K., MacRae, N., & Sladyk, K. [2014]. *Occupational therapy essentials for clinical competence* [2nd ed.]. Thorofare, NJ: SLACK Incorporated; 590.)

Case Study #3

The OT shares with you the plan for supporting the trustworthiness of the current study. Now that you have several weeks of experience with the meal preparation group, you are invited to contribute your reflections and ideas. A manual is being written with guidelines for conducting the intervention and specific instructions for administering the surveys and scoring the observational check sheet. This will help ensure consistency in the program and the assessment of participants. The two of you brainstorm about ways to improve the manual. You agree that your role will be to assist with running the program and administering the surveys. Also, both you and the OT will fill out a check sheet for each participant as a way of cross-checking observations.

Case Study #4

When the OT conducted the initial literature search prior to designing the meal preparation group program, an appropriate PICO for this search might be:

- For individuals between 18 and 85 years of age who have cognitive and/or physical functional deficits, does a group program involving meal preparation improve socialization, confidence, and independent living skills compared with group rehabilitation programs that do not include meal preparation?

MAKING EVIDENCE-BASED DECISIONS

Knowledge of research designs and an understanding of what constitutes rigorous investigation will enhance any occupational therapy scholarly endeavor. In addition to providing a framework for developing an original study, this knowledge underscores the critical appraisal of published research literature, which is essential for making evidence-based practice decisions. There are a number of sources that offer specific detailed guidelines for scholarly practice, or evidence-based practice—for example, Kielhofner (2006), Taylor (2007), and Melnyk and Fineout-Overholt (2011). This process begins when a clinical situation or problem is encountered in which not all the needed information is at hand. Then inquiry proceeds as a series of steps (Lin, Murphy, & Robinson, 2010).

In step 1, an occupational therapy practitioner seeking specific knowledge to guide clinical decision making formulates a clear, sufficiently focused, answerable clinical question. PICO or PICOT (Melnyk & Fineout-Overholt, 2011) is the acronym for a practical structured approach to framing clinical questions pertinent to the care of a specific client or a category of clients seen routinely. *P* refers to the person, problem, or population of interest; *I* to the issue or intervention being considered; *C* to a comparison such as an alternate intervention or no intervention; *O* to the outcome that would be affected by the intervention; and *T* to a time frame. Here are two examples:

- For adolescents with clinical depression receiving antidepressant medication (P), what is the effect of a group occupational therapy program (I) consisting of biweekly 1-hour sessions over 4 weeks (T) on participation in the community (O) compared with antidepressant medication alone (C)?

- For elders 65 and older with a history of falls who are living at home (P), does in-home fall prevention education by an occupational therapist (I) result in lower incidence of falls in the home (O) compared with outpatient clinic–based occupational therapy fall prevention education (C) at 6-month follow-up (T)?

The PICO or PICOT system prompts the occupational therapy practitioner to formulate a clinical question that supports an effective systematic search of the published literature for directly related research evidence, which is step 2 in the evidence-based practice process. Up-to-date published peer-reviewed studies can be located via Internet sources such as Google Scholar or SpringerLink or the electronic database search system of a college or university library. Electronic databases applicable to occupational therapy practice range from specialized compilations (e.g., OTseeker; Bennett et al., 2003)—to broad-based compilations of thousands of journals, including *EBSCOhost, CINAHL, Medline/PubMed,* and *PsychINFO.* Collected systematic reviews and meta-analyses are published in the Cochrane Library database. Working collaboratively with colleagues to locate sources is also worthwhile. The practitioner typically begins the search for relevant literature by using keywords suggested by the clinical question. However, search terms must sometimes be adapted to the standardized medical vocabulary used by some electronic databases. Fortunately, there are several excellent resources that teach the often arduous process of searching the literature and accessing pertinent research articles (Kielhofner, 2006; Melnyk & Fineout-Overholt, 2011; Taylor, 2007).

Step 3 is *critical appraisal of the evidence.* The occupational therapy practitioner carefully assesses the quality and trustworthiness of the research evidence in the published literature that has the most direct bearing on the clinical question. Once an article relevant to the clinical question is found in a peer-reviewed journal, it is important to consider the type of research design and whether it is quantitative or qualitative, the purpose of investigation and research questions or hypotheses, the nature of the study participants, the independent and dependent variables, how the dependent variables were measured, the methods that were used to administer the intervention and/or gather the data, and the authors' findings. Useful guidelines for critical review of quantitative and qualitative research, prepared by the McMaster University Occupational Therapy Evidence-Based Practice Research Group, can be retrieved from the Internet (Law et al., 1998a, 1998b; Letts et al., 2007a, 2007b).

Once the available evidence has been critically appraised, in step 4 the occupational therapy practitioner draws an unbiased conclusion, based on integration of information from the multiple studies, as to how the evidence answered the clinical question. This action, sometimes called formulating the "clinical bottom line" (Kielhofner, 2006, p. 680), is followed by step 5, in which the practitioner integrates the answer to the clinical question with his or her clinical expertise and considers the values, preferences, and unique situation of the client or client group to make a decision regarding the most suitable intervention (Dijkers, Murphy, & Krellman, 2012). Finally, in step 6, the practitioner evaluates the outcome of the clinical decision.

CONCLUSION

Scholarship and scholarly practice are essential for the professional growth of any occupational therapy practitioner, as well as for developing the knowledge base of the discipline of occupational therapy. Understanding the types of quantitative and qualitative research designs and their suitable applications, as well as determinants of what constitutes rigorous investigation, is needed to support both research and evidence-based practice. Finding the evidence needed for clinical decision making entails following a series of steps, from formulating a question to integrating the results of a focused literature search into practice. In any occupational therapy scholarly endeavor, collaboration is a key to narrowing the gap between the new knowledge gained from research and its implementation in everyday practice settings.

SUGGESTED WEBSITES

- American Occupational Therapy Foundation: www.aotf.org
- Cochrane Collaboration: http://www.cochrane.org/cochrane-reviews/about-cochrane-library
- National Guideline Clearinghouse: http://www.guideline.gov/

REVIEW QUESTIONS

1. What is the distinction between scholarship and scholarly practice?

    a. There is no distinction.

    b. Scholarship refers to research, while scholarly practice refers to evidence-based practice.

    c. Scholarship has to do with reading published evidence, while scholarly practice has to do with conducting research and publishing the evidence.

    d. Scholarship is associated with purely academic study or achievement, while scholarly practice is the responsibility of OT practitioners.

2. How can one distinguish between quantitative and qualitative research?

    a. Qualitative research is always exploratory and descriptive, while quantitative research is never exploratory or descriptive.

    b. Quantitative researchers gather data that are based on numbers, while qualitative researchers gather data that are based on language.

    c. Qualitative research is driven by the perspectives of the participants, while quantitative research is driven by the perspectives of the investigators.

    d. Both b and c are true.

3. Why are outcome studies often called quasi-experimental?

    a. Unlike experimental research, outcome studies do not include independent and dependent variables.

    b. Outcome studies may lack some or all of the features of true experimental studies, namely prospective design, a control group, randomization, and blinding.

    c. Outcome studies cannot quantitatively demonstrate the impact of an intervention on a population of interest.

    d. In outcome research, the investigators do not manipulate any conditions experienced by the study participants.

4. In the hierarchical system for classifying levels of evidence, what type of research is placed at the apex of the two-dimensional pyramid as representing the strongest level of evidence?

    a. Longitudinal research

    b. Randomized controlled trials

    c. Descriptive studies

    d. Outcome research

5. Which of the following best completes the sentence? Research validity, also called rigor or trustworthiness:

    a. Is a consideration only in experimental research methodology.

    b. Is an indication that the research reflects actual phenomena in the world.

    c. Entails embedding sound principles and practices—agreed on by the scientific community—into every step of a research process.

    d. Both b and c.

6. PICO, the acronym for a practical structured approach to framing clinical questions, stands for:

    a. Program, individual, computation, output

    b. Procedure, idea, client, outgrowth

    c. Person, intervention, comparison, outcome

    d. Both a and c.

7. In a systematic search of the published literature providing research evidence directly related to the clinical question, suitable articles cannot be located:

    a. On electronic databases such as PubMed

    b. Using Internet sources such as Google Scholar or OTseeker

    c. In magazines and newspapers

    d. Via collaboration with colleagues

8. Once a research article relevant to the guiding clinical question is located in a peer-reviewed journal, what is the next step?

    a. Conduct a critical analysis to assess the quality and trustworthiness of the research evidence.

    b. Integrate the results of the critical analysis into the intervention.

    c. Come to a conclusion as to how the evidence in the article answers the clinical question.

    d. Read the article in its entirety.

9. The counterparts to the trustworthiness criterion of truth value in qualitative and quantitative research perspectives are:

    a. Credibility and internal validity, respectively

    b. Transferability and external validity, respectively

    c. Dependability and reliability, respectively

    d. Confirmability and objectivity, respectively

10. The counterparts to the trustworthiness criterion of consistency in qualitative and quantitative research perspectives are

    a. Credibility and internal validity, respectively

    b. Transferability and external validity, respectively

    c. Dependability and reliability, respectively

    d. Confirmability and objectivity, respectively

REFERENCES

American Occupational Therapy Association. (n.d.a). *Guidelines to critically appraised paper (CAP) worksheet evidence exchange.* Retrieved from https://www.aota.org/-/media/Corporate/Files/Practice/EvidenceExchange/CAP%20Guidelines%20for%20Evidence%20Exchange.pdf

American Occupational Therapy Association. (n.d.b) Guidelines to critically appraised paper (CAP) worksheet evidence exchange. Retrieved from https://www.aota.org/-/media/Corporate/Files/Practice/EvidenceExchange/CAP%20Guidelines%20for%20Evidence%20Exchange.pdf

American Occupational Therapy Association. (2009). Scholarship in occupational therapy. *American Journal of Occupational Therapy 63*(6), 790-796.

Bennett, S., Hoffman, T., McCluskey, A., McKenna, K., Strong, J., & Tooth, L. (2003). Introducing OTseeker (Occupational Therapy Systematic Evaluation of Evidence): A new evidence database for occupational therapists. *American Journal of Occupational Therapy, 57*(6), 635-638.

Christiansen, C., & Lou, J. Q. (2001). Ethical considerations related to evidence-based practice. *American Journal of Occupational Therapy, 55*(3), 345-349.

Cook, J. V. (2001). *Qualitative research in occupational therapy: Strategies and experiences.* San Diego, CA: Singular Publishing.

Cooper, H., Hedges, L. V., & Valentine, J. C. (2009). *The handbook of research synthesis and meta-analysis* (2nd ed.). New York: Russell Sage Foundation.

Dijkers, M. P., Murphy, S. L., & Krellman, J. (2012). Evidence-based practice for rehabilitation professionals: Concepts and controversies. *Archives of Physical Medicine and Rehabilitation, 93*(8), S164-S176.

Guba, E. G. (1981). ERIC/ECTJ annual review paper: Criteria for assessing the trustworthiness of naturalistic inquiries. *Educational Communication and Technology Journal, 29*(2), 75-91.

Haertlein, C., & Coppard, B. M. (2003). Scholarship and occupational therapy (2003 concept paper). *American Journal of Occupational Therapy, 57*(6), 641-643.

Holm, M. B. (2000). The 2000 Eleanor Clarke Slagle Lecture. Our mandate for the new millennium: Evidence-based practice. *American Journal of Occupational Therapy, 54*(6), 575-585.

Kielhofner, G. (1982a). Qualitative research: Part two. Methodological approaches and relevance to occupational therapy. *OTJR: Occupation, Participation and Health, 2*(3), 150-170.

Kielhofner, G. (1982b). Qualitative research: Part one. Paradigmatic grounds and issues of reliability. *OTJR: Occupation, Participation and Health, 2*(2), 67-79.

Kielhofner, G. (2006). *Research in occupational therapy: Methods of inquiry for enhancing practice.* Philadelphia: F. A. Davis Company.

Krefting, L. (1991). Rigor in qualitative research: The assessment of trustworthiness. *American Journal of Occupational Therapy, 45*(3), 214-222.

Law, M., & MacDermid, J. (2008). *Evidence-based rehabilitation: A guide to practice.* Thorofare, NJ: SLACK Incorporated.

Law, M., Stewart, D., Pollock, N., Letts, L., Bosch, J., & Westmorland, M. (1998a). *Guidelines for critical review form: Quantitative studies.* Retrieved from http://www.srs-mcmaster.ca/Portals/20/pdf/ebp/quanguidelines.pdf

Law, M., Stewart, D., Pollock, N., Letts, L., Bosch, J., & Westmorland, M. (1998b). *Critical review form: Quantitative studies.* Retrieved from http://www.srs-mcmaster.ca/Portals/20/pdf/ebp/quanreview.pdf

Letts, L., Wilkins, S., Law, M., Stewart, D., Bosch, J., & Westmorland, M. (2007a). *Guidelines for critical review form: Qualitative studies.* Retrieved from http://www.srs-mcmaster.ca/Portals/20/pdf/ebp/qualguidelines_version2.0.pdf

Letts, L., Wilkins, S., Law, M., Stewart, D., Bosch, J., & Westmorland, M. (2007b). *Critical review form: Qualitative studies.* Retrieved from http://www.srs-mcmaster.ca/Portals/20/pdf/ebp/qualreview_version2.0.pdf

Lin, S. H., Murphy, S. L., & Robinson, J. C. (2010) Facilitating evidence-based practice: Process, strategies and resources. *American Journal of Occupational Therapy, 64*(1), 164-171.

Littleton, A. G. (2013, May 20). In the kitchen. Promoting socialization, confidence and independent living skills as part of a food preparation group. *OT Practice, 18*(9), 7-11.

Mack, N., Woodsong, C., MacQueen, K. M., Guest, G., & Namey, E. (2005). *Qualitative research methods: A data collector's field guide.* Research Triangle Park, NC: Family Health International. Retrieved from http://www.fhi360.org/resource/qualitative-research-methods-data-collectors-field-guide

Melnyk, B., and Fineout-Overholt, E. (2011). *Evidence-based practice in nursing & healthcare: A guide to best practice* (2nd ed.). Riverwoods, IL: Wolters Kluwer Health/Lippincott Williams & Wilkins.

Merrill, S. C. (1985). Qualitative methods in occupational therapy research: An application. *OTJR: Occupation, Participation and Health, 5*(4), 209-222.

Mortenson, W. B., & Oliffe, J. L. (2009). Mixed methods research in occupational therapy: A survey and critique. *OTJR: Occupation, Participation and Health, 29*(1), 14-23.

Ottenbacher, K. J., and Hinderer, S. R. (2001). Evidence-based practice: Methods to evaluate individual patient improvement. *American Journal of Physical Medicine and Rehabilitation, 80*(10), 786-796.

Papadimitriou, C., Magasi, S., & Frank, G. (2012). Current thinking in qualitative research: Evidence-based practice, moral philosophies, and political struggle. *OTJR: Occupation, Participation and Health, 32*(1 Suppl. 1), S2-S5.

Sackett, D. L., Rosenberg, W. M. C., Gray, J. A. M., Haynes, R. B., & Richardson, W. S. (1996). Evidence based medicine: What it is and what it isn't. *British Medical Journal, 312*(7023), 71-72.

Taylor, M. C. (2007). *Evidence-based practice for occupational therapists* (2nd ed.). Malden, MA: Blackwell Publishing.

Tickle-Degnan, L. (1999). Organizing, evaluating, and using evidence in occupational therapy practice. *American Journal of Occupational Therapy, 53*(5), 537-539.

Wholey, J. S., Hatry, H. P., & Newcomer, K. E. (2010). *Handbook of practical program evaluation* (3rd ed.). San Francisco: John Wiley & Sons.

Financial Disclosures

Dr. Karen Brady has no financial or proprietary interest in the materials presented herein.

Dr. Lisa Burns has no financial or proprietary interest in the materials presented herein.

Dr. Nancy W. Doyle has no financial or proprietary interest in the materials presented herein.

Kimberly Erler has no financial or proprietary interest in the materials presented herein.

Dr. Karen Jacobs receives royalties from AOTA, IOS Press, Elsevier, and SLACK Incorporated; a grant from National Institute on Disability and Rehabilitation Research; and she is on the executive council and Chair of one of the technical committees for Human Factors and Ergonomics Society.

Brenda Kennell has no financial or proprietary interest in the materials presented herein.

Barbara Larson has no financial or proprietary interest in the materials presented herein.

Ann McCullough has no financial or proprietary interest in the materials presented herein.

Sarah McKinnon has no financial or proprietary interest in the materials presented herein.

Dr. Julie Ann Nastasi has no financial or proprietary interest in the materials presented herein.

Dr. Linda Niemeyer has no financial or proprietary interest in the materials presented herein.

Melissa J. Tilton has no financial or proprietary interest in the materials presented herein.

Christi Vicino reviews books for Wolters Kluwer.

Index

Printed in the United States
by Baker & Taylor Publisher Services